D1072526

EUGLENA

DISTRIBUTED BY
The Rutgers University Press
New Brunswick, New Jersey

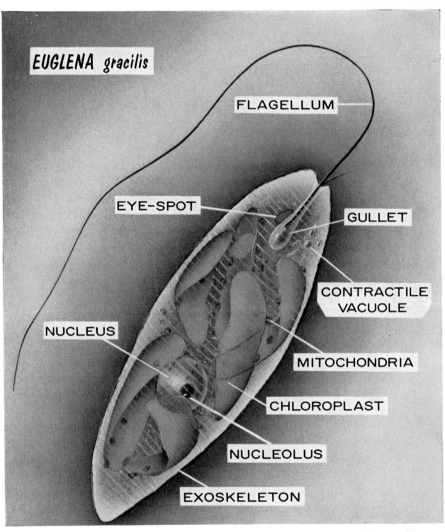

Schematized *Euglena gracilis* cell indicating its general structure and organelles.

EUGLENA

An Experimental Organism for Biochemical and Biophysical Studies

JEROME J. WOLKEN

Biophysical Research Laboratory, Eye and Ear Hospital,
University of Pittsburgh School of Medicine,
Pittsburgh, Pennsylvania

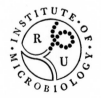

INSTITUTE OF MICROBIOLOGY

Rutgers, The State University   1961

Library of Congress Catalog Card Number: 61-10481

This volume is one of a series
of studies in microbiology
published by
The Institute of Microbiology
at Rutgers, The State University
and distributed by the
Rutgers University Press

Printed in the United States of America
by the Quinn & Boden Company, Inc., Rahway, New Jersey

Dedicated to
The Memory of
D. O. M. W.

PREFACE

To find out how—and why—light affects the growth, structure, and photoreceptor systems of plants and animals, I began with a unicellular protozoan flagellate, *Euglena*. These studies were initiated at the Rockefeller Institute for Medical Research during the tenure of an American Cancer Society Fellowship (1951-1952) and have been continuously pursued at the Biophysical Research Laboratory, Eye and Ear Hospital, University of Pittsburgh School of Medicine.

Euglena is ideally suited for such experimental studies because of its dramatic behavior as an *animal*-like cell in the dark and a *plant* cell in the light. An active photosynthetic *Euglena* in the light is green, in the dark it becomes "colorless;" when restored to the light again, it becomes green in a few hours. The light ↔ dark phenomena are accompanied by morphological and chemical changes of the organism. The experiments to be described were designed to get at a molecular basis for cellular structure and function—then to see how far these results could apply to the problems common to photosynthesis, phototropism, vision, and communication.

No systematic attempt will be made to discuss the classification and idiosyncrasies of the many species of *Euglena;* this has been done by M. Gojdics (*The Genus Euglena,* 1953) and E. G. Pringsheim (*Contributions Toward a Monograph on the Genus Euglena,* 1956). Nor have I attempted to cover metabolic matters already reviewed in Volumes I and II of *The Biochemistry and Physiology of Protozoa* (eds. Lwoff, and Lwoff and Hutner). To those interested in the broader aspects of photosynthesis and photoreception, reference is made to

viii   *Preface*

Photosynthesis and Related Processes, Volume I, and parts 1 and 2 of Volume II, by E. Rabinowitch; the Brookhaven Symposium on *The Photochemical Apparatus: Its Structure and Function* (1959); the New York Academy of Sciences conference on *Photoreception* (1958), and to the many recent symposia, reviews, and current journal literature.

This book is primarily concerned with the use of *Euglena* in studying photoreception; it is also hoped that biologists, biochemists, and biophysicists will find in *Euglena* a remarkably versatile research tool for attacking some of their problems.

I would like to thank Drs. S. H. Hutner and L. Provasoli of the Haskins Laboratories for introducing me to *Euglena* as an exceptional experimental "animal," as well as for many stimulating discussions and continued enthusiasm. I am indebted to Drs. G. E. Palade and K. R. Porter of the Rockefeller Institute in whose laboratories these researches began. I should like to express my appreciation to Dr. M. F. McCaslin, to the McClintic Endowment, and to the administrative staff of the Eye and Ear Hospital for providing laboratory facilities and for continual research support. I especially would like to thank all of my colleagues who have worked with me at some time in the laboratory and shared with me the pleasures and anxieties in doing the experiments.

Thanks are also due to the United States Public Health Service and to the National Council to Combat Blindness, Inc., who have given sustained support, not only through financial help, but even more through their continuous interest and encouragement to attack the problem of photoreception in its broader sense.

For their patience in typing and retyping, my thanks to Mrs. M. Rozen and Mrs. R. Engelmore, who have seen this book from its beginnings, and to Mr. L. Mastro for his skill in converting many of the sketches into drawings. Finally, the editorial assistance of Mr. R. A Day of the Institute of Microbiology is gratefully acknowledged.

For their financial support in making this publication possible, I would like to express my deep gratitude to Mr. Ross E. Willis, to Dr. Selman A. Waksman and the Foundation for Microbiology; and to the Institute of Microbiology, Rutgers, The State University.

JEROME J. WOLKEN

ACKNOWLEDGMENTS

I am obliged to the editors of *Biochimica et Biophysica Acta,* the *Journal of Cellular and Comparative Physiology,* the *Journal of General Physiology,* the *Journal of Protozoology, Nature, Science,* and the *Transactions* and *Annals of the New York Academy of Sciences* for permission to reprint various figures, and to quote from our papers in these journals. Thanks are also due to the publishers of *New Biology* for permission to reproduce, in part, Figs. 2 and 3.

CONTENTS

EUGLENA

1 INTRODUCTION

"In research dealing with physics, chemistry, and physiology, one always attempts to isolate relatively simple systems, and to determine their exact conditions." (Alexis Carrel—*Man The Unknown*, p. 50, Harper and Brothers, New York, 1935.)

The mechanism of energy conversion, transfer, and storage in living systems is one of the greatest challenges for research. This underlies the problems of how organisms reproduce, move, photosynthesize, see, and react in an integrated fashion, *i.e.*, as a whole organism.

The choice of the experimental "animal" in biological research is often decisive; it should not be a casual matter. Simple practicality is all-important at the start. Is the organism easy to keep and hardy in the laboratory? Does it grow vigorously? Can its chemical (nutritional) and physical (temperature, light, pressure, etc.) environment be controlled easily? What are its responses; are they easily measurable? Tissue cells and unicellular microorganisms—especially the photosynthetic bacteria and algae—are attractive and have been used with great success in attacking some of these problems. Recent advances in nutrition enable us to grow many of these cells and organisms in completely defined media, so providing a large population of cells for experimental studies. It also permits analysis of the effects of the chemical and physical environment on the mass populations as well as on individual organisms or cells. Bacteria, protozoa, and algae, within their small confines, undertake the same functions with their *organelles* as the higher plant or animal with its billions of cells. For instance, certain cell components, the mitochondria, are comparable to "organs" in higher plants and animals in the sense that they are functionally specialized. There is, however, a great difference in the level of functional integration achieved in the "organelle" as compared to the "organ": it is much simpler in the former, still "biochemical," not yet physiological. Yet, within the small structure of these organelles, the same functions are carried out.

When one speaks of microorganisms, one generally thinks of bacteria, yeasts, and viruses, but unicellular organisms also include algae, protozoa, and many fungi. *Euglena* is a unicellular protozoan, more accurately an "algal flagellate"; it has the characteristics of a plant but shares as well some of the attributes of an animal cell. Lwoff (83) says it is impossible to give a satisfactory definition of protozoa. Hutner thinks of "true" protozoa as the particle-ingesting protists. Protista is the inclusive term for *all* non or acellular ("unicellular") organisms.

The morphology, physiology, and biochemistry of the euglenoids have been reviewed by Jahn (62, 63) and more recently by Lwoff, Hutner, and Provasoli in Volumes I and II of *Biochemistry and Physiology of Protozoa*. In some respects, knowledge of the chemistry of protists is primitive. Some of the green (photosynthetic) flagellates thrive in simple media, and have greatly advanced these studies.

Organisms range from *autotrophic* (thriving on minerals alone) to *heterotrophic* (needing organic substances). When Lwoff and Dusi (83-86) at the Pasteur Institute discovered that certain chlorophyll-bearing euglenas need organic growth factors, the old definition of "autotroph" had to be revised. Some of these considerations will be taken up in the discussion on the comparative aspects of photosynthesis. Classically, in T. H. Huxley's definition, animals are denoted as those forms of life which require pre-formed organic molecules in their nutrition, and which possess such characteristics as locomotion, flexible cell walls, and some sort of integrated "nervous" control, all in response to their reliance on ingested particulate food. Photosynthetic plants, in contrast, depend far less on externally supplied organic substances; they can synthesize all or nearly all their constituents from inorganic molecules, which implies that the hallmark of animality is the ingestion of particulate food. This seems a more direct link with "protozoa" construed as "proto-zoa," *i.e., first* or *true* animals. Some distinctions between the "plants" and the "animals" are shown in Table 1. These definitions tend to lessen the embarrassments felt by many botanists in dealing with fungi and bacteria, and by zoologists in dealing with algal flagellates.

TABLE 1

SOME DISTINCTIONS BETWEEN PLANTS AND ANIMALS

	Plants	Animals
Energy source	Photosynthesis	Organic material
Chlorophyll	Generally present (except in fungi)	Absent (except in some particle-ingesting flagellates)
Principal reserve food	Starch, oil (in some)	Glycogen, fat
External foodstuff	Absorbed osmotically	Ingested
Active movement	Restricted (except for some flagellates and the gametes of plant cells)	Usually present
Cell walls	Generally rigid (except in some flagellates)	Generally flexible
Nervous system	Absent	Present (an equivalent presumably present in protozoa)

General Characteristics of Euglena

The class *Euglenineae* or *Euglenophyta* (the name derived from *Euglena*) is a natural taxonomic group within the flagellates. There is a remote, though definite, relationship to the green algae; the *Euglenaceae*, the *Euglenineae* with photosynthetic pigments, are the only other organisms containing, like the *Chlorophyceae* and higher plants, chlorophyll *b* in addition to chlorophyll *a*. Some euglenas are colorless; others are green, red, yellow, or brown. In three recent monographs by Pringsheim (113), Gojdics (39), and Grell (49), the many species of *Euglena* are defined in detail. More than 150 species are recognized.

Euglena has presented a problem of classification to taxonomists, ill at ease with protists, for they embody features commonly and uncritically denoted as "plant-" or "animal-like." It has been speculated that euglenas may have been close to the origins of the higher plants and most fungi; the euglenoid flagellates are probably remote from the flagellates that are supposed to have given rise to the cellular animals (*i.e.*, metazoa), as shown in Fig. 1. The abundance of question marks

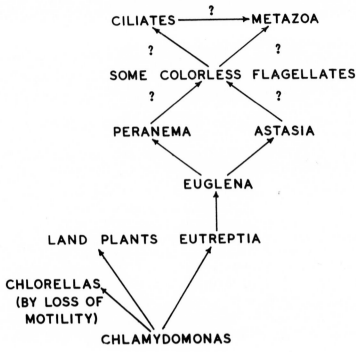

Fig. 1. Affinities of the green flagellates.

in the figure indicates the primitiveness of knowledge of the affinities among protozoan groups, and their kinship to the metazoa. Hutner and Provasoli look upon the algal flagellates as a heterogeneous group occupying a central position along lines of plant → animal descent (59, 60). From the scheme in Fig. 1, it will be noted that *Chlamydomonas* → land plant lines go back to green algae. The green algae, in turn, go back to *Chlamydomonas*. This is inferred from the fact that the sex cells (gametes) of multicellular or filamentous green algae are very *Chlamydomonas*-like. Fresh water ponds and the oceans have a wealth of *Chlamydomonas* and closely related flagellates. It should be noted that these green-pigmented forms are sharply different from brown-pigmented flagellates, whose affinities are more to the brown seaweeds and diatoms.

Euglena is a classical organism that every student of biology has observed. Euglenas are ubiquitous in fresh-water bodies. They favor waters rich in organic materials, and some species favor damp soils; the closely related *Eutreptia* is common in the ocean near cities. In the sense of adaptability to laboratory conditions, *Euglena gracilis* is the weed among the photosynthetic euglenoids, and the Z strain is among the very hardiest.

An active, swimming *E. gracilis* is elongated, 50×15 μ, and is sometimes as large as 70×20 μ. It has a helicoidally striated limiting membrane with barely visible ridges. From a "gullet" or cytopharynx protrudes the whipping flagellum. *E. gracilis* has many discoid chloroplasts, a single conspicuous nucleus (seen as a central and somewhat anterior clear area), numerous mitochondria, vacuoles, granules, and lipid inclusions. Among the inclusions is a tight orange-red pigmented group which comprises the stigma or *eyespot*, situated close to the gullet. An active *Euglena* is schematized in Fig. 2, and in Fig. 3 it is compared with other flagellated organisms. In an actual photomicrograph at low magnification (Fig. 4), many of the structures of *E. gracilis* can easily be identified.

Application of powerful electron microscopes and other specialized instruments to explore the morphology of *Euglena* has venerable antecedents. In 1675, Antony van Leeuwenhoek probably first described the euglenas (21):

"These animalcules had diverse colors, some being whitish and transparent; others with green and very glittering scales; others again were green. . . . And the motion of most of these animalcules in the water was so swift, and so various, upwards, downwards, and round about, that 'twas wonderful to see. . . ."

Euglena grown under light in the laboratory is beautifully green and concentrates toward the light. Its greenness comes from chlorophyll in chloroplasts. (The *Euglena* pigments as they pertain to the structure and photochemistry of the chloroplast are further elaborated in Chapters 3 to 6.) In the dark, cultures have both motile and quiescent forms. Many are rounded-up, reduced in size, and obviously lacking or low in chlorophyll. Rounded-up organisms encased in cell-wall slime are called *palmelloid*. These inactive or sluggish forms possess less distinct organelles. Ability to assume the slender "gracilis" form is favored by light and by fresh culture media, especially dilute media. Active swimming, as distinguished from crawling movements and body distortions ("metaboly"), is resumed, along with chlorophyll synthesis, when they are restored to light.

Since *Euglena* can be profoundly different in structure and chemistry depending on whether it is grown in light or darkness, it is an ideal organism for studying the gross structural changes as well as

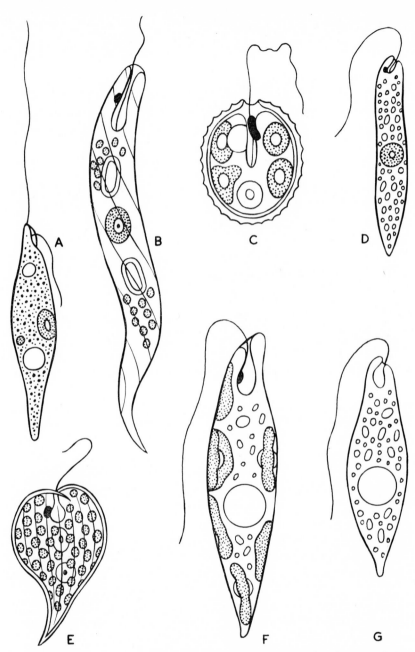

Fig. 2. Various shapes and sizes of the Euglenoids. Reproduced in part from
F. W. Jane, "Famous Plant-Animal, *Euglena*," *New Biology*, 19:114 (1955).
A. *Heteronema acus;* B. *Euglena spirogyra;* C. *Trachelomonas hispida;* D.
Astasia longa; E. *Phacus pleuronectes;* F. *Euglena gracilis* (light-grown); G.
Euglena gracilis (dark-grown).

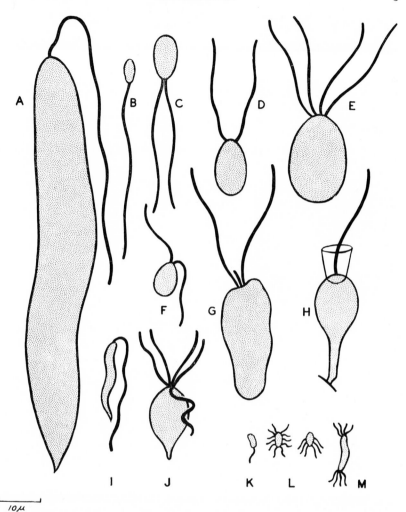

10μ

Fig. 3. Variety of flagellated organisms (76). A. *Euglena gracilis* (green). B. *Echinus,* spermatozoid of a sea urchin. C. *Scourfeldia* (green) with posterior flagella. D. *Chlamydomonas* (green) with anterior flagella. E. *Carteria* (green) closely related to *Chlamydomonas.* F. *Saprolegnia,* zoospore of aquatic fungus. G. *Pyrmnesium* (orange). H. *Codonosiga* (protozoan). I. *Trypanosoma* (parasitic protozoan). J. *Trichomonas* (parasitic flagellate). K. *Vibrio cholerae* (bacterium). L. *Salmonella typhi.* M. *Rhodospirillum* (red photosynthetic bacterium).

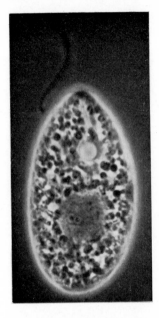

Fig. 4. Photomicrograph of light-grown *Euglena*, 1600×.

the underlying chemistry in a living cell—above all the chloroplast and its pigments—during the light ↔ dark transformations.

Fig. 2 shows some other euglenas to indicate the variety of sizes, shapes, and structures in the group. Jahn (64) and Gojdics (39) illustrated a considerable number of euglenoids in great detail. The photosynthetic euglenoids comprise a bizarre variety of forms, and no doubt their physiological specializations, when uncovered, will prove to be equally bizarre. We have studied several strains and varieties of *Euglena*, including the achlorophyllous *Astasia* as well as the chlorophyllous Z strain of *E. gracilis* and *E. granulata;* but unless otherwise noted, *Euglena gracilis* var. *bacillaris* is referred to in the text.

How does structure condition the function of a given organelle? In our experiments, *Euglena*'s structures were viewed as expressing function: *e.g.,* how does the chloroplast structure at a molecular level determine its functions in the photosynthesizing cell? In teleological language, how does the eyespot help the organism to detect light? How does the structure of the flagella enable the organism to swim swiftly and surely toward the light? How does the eyespot influence flagellar behavior? Our experiments were designed in an attempt to answer such questions; they will be described, beginning with those having to do with the structure of the organism, then going on to the photoreceptors (chloroplast and eyespot), the pigments, and the effects of light, temperature, drugs, and metals on its chemistry and structure.

Growth Characteristics of Euglena

The organism divides in two upon reaching a certain size and maturity; sexual reproduction is unknown. Nuclear and cytoplasmic division take place. Division necessarily is complicated: not alone the nucleus, but also the organelles (chloroplasts, eyespot, flagella), are independently self-reproducing, or at least, do not lose their identity during division. Leedale (75), who studied nuclear division in 32 species of the Euglenaceae from 13 genera, observed true mitosis, but it differed from the "classical" form in that the endosome of the nucleus persists throughout mitosis, dividing as a structure distinct from the chromosome. He also noted that *E. gracilis* had 45 chromosomes and that mitosis lasted from 2 to 5 hours, of which anaphase took from 35 to 86 minutes. This is slow when compared with other organisms and tissues in which anaphase takes from 1 to 20 minutes.

Rate studies on cultures are good for discerning relations between growth, *i.e.*, number of cells, and environmental factors, especially kinds and concentrations of nutrients. This is best done in a medium with all ingredients known. In the growth or log phase, all the organisms are dividing regularly. Growth curves for *Euglena* are now accurately reproducible. A typical growth curve is reproduced in Fig. 5. The increments in mass of *Euglena* are now measured spectrophotometrically at a wavelength (750 mμ) where there is little interference from the chlorophyll pigments. In the earlier work, actual counts of the number of organisms were carried out. Chiefly responsible for this reproducibility in growth is the control over the environmental conditions; also, we were dealing with large numbers of organisms, and so, as in other like microbiological situations, individual variability becomes statistically negligible.

Few species of *Euglena* have been cultivated pure. As noted, *E. gracilis* is a hardy laboratory weed among the euglenas. A simple synthetic liquid medium of the composition indicated in Table 2 was devised by Hutner and Provasoli for batch or continuous cultivation of *E. gracilis*. This medium was used for all studies on *E. gracilis* var. *bacillaris*. Variations in the media were carried out to test the effect on growth and pigment synthesis. (See Appendix for a description of

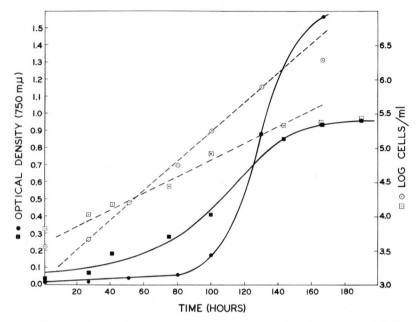

Fig. 5. Typical growth curve: optical density versus time (——— ● ——— light-grown; ——— ■ ——— dark-grown); log of the number of cells per millimeter versus time in hours during log phase of growth only, slope of which was used to determine growth rate (---- ⊙ ---- light-grown; ---- ▣ ---- dark-grown).

a richer organic medium to elicit faster and denser growth and for other culture media for *Euglena*.)

Hutner, Provasoli, Pringsheim, and others have shaped *Euglena* and many protozoan forms into important tools in nutritional research; their findings have cleared the way to investigations of the metabolism of *Euglena*. Let us consider the nutrition of *Euglena*. Unlike land plants, *Euglena* cannot utilize nitrates; it will grow rapidly if given ammonia supplemented with amino acids. *E. gracilis* is known as one of the acetate flagellates, generally preferring acids and alcohols to sugars as their main carbon source; this is a nutritional pattern quite unlike familiar green algae, such as *Chlorella,* and the land plants, whose favorite external substrate is glucose or sucrose. Since *Euglena* can grow rapidly on acetate as the sole substrate, it must have some means of making Krebs-cycle intermediates from acetate. In land plants, acetate can be converted to carbohydrate via the "glyoxylic acid shunt." Since *E. gracilis* can utilize glycolic and lactic acids in media of low pH (<4.0), it is likely that *Euglena* may have a highly

TABLE 2

STANDARD MEDIUM FOR GROWTH OF *Euglena gracilis*

	g/l
KH_2PO_4	0.5
$MgSO_4 \cdot 7H_2O$	0.5
L-Glutamic acid	5.0
DL-Malic acid	1.0
$CaCO_3$	0.1
$(NH_4)_6Mo_7O_{24} \cdot 4H_2O$	0.010
Thiamine·HCl (Vitamin B_1)	0.001
Cyanocobalamin (Vitamin B_{12})	1×10^{-6}
"Metals 36"	

One ml of metals' solution per 100 ml of medium.

Metals 36	g/l
Ethylenediaminetetraacetic acid	5.0
$MnSO_4 \cdot H_2O$	6.15
$ZnSO_4 \cdot 7H_2O$	11.0
$FeSO_4(NH_4)_2SO_4 \cdot 6H_2O$	1.75
$CoSO_4 \cdot 7H_2O$	0.286
$CuSO_4 \cdot 5H_2O$	0.039
H_3BO_3	0.028
KI	0.0012

pH of final medium—3.3 to 3.6.

developed glyoxylic acid entry to the Krebs cycle (58); *Euglena* diverges from land plants in respect to vitamins: it absolutely needs vitamin B_{12}. Indeed *Euglena* is widely used to measure vitamin B_{12}. Thiamine (vitamin B_1) is also required.

Euglena in light photosynthesizes like an orthodox plant, but has a peculiar carbohydrate as an end product—paramylum—which hydrolyzes to glucose. Metabolic patterns like *Euglena*'s are common in protists, *e.g.*, the aerobic photosynthetic bacteria are nutritionally not very different, even to needing vitamins. As noted, while *Euglena* can photosynthesize, it does not have to. To produce carbohydrates from CO_2 and H_2O it requires light, of course, both for synthesis of pigments and as an energy source. When deprived of light, *Euglena* can grow with unimpaired vigor in certain substrate-rich media. Though capable of using simple sugars in certain media, it can also grow well on simpler organic compounds, such as ethanol or acetate.

Euglenas have been continuously maintained in our laboratory, in the culture medium listed in Table 2, at room temperature (25°C) either with continuous light (300 ft candles) or in complete darkness. They have been kept in cotton-plugged 1-liter bottles containing 330 ml of nutrient fluid, or in 30-ml test tubes containing 10 ml of nu-

TABLE 3

Comparative Growth Rates of Various Organisms in Terms of $\log_{10}$ Units per Day

Organism		k	Conditions
Bacteria	*Escherichia coli* *	26.0	lactose broth
	Pseudomonas fluorescens *	13.0	glucose broth
	Azotobacter chroococcum *	6.0	urea, glucose
		1.3	sugar, mineral salts
Yeast	*Willia anomala* *	6.0	glucose, yeast extract
Protozoa	*Tetrahymena geleii* *	1.8	yeast autolysate
Algae	*Anabaena cylindrica* *	0.32	light, CO_2, NO_3^-
	Chlorella pyrenoidosa *	0.85	light, CO_2, NO_3^-
		0.40	dark, glucose, NO_3^-
		0.21	dark, acetate, NO_3^-
	Chlorella vulgaris *	0.49	light, glucose, NH_4NO_3
		0.29	dark, glucose, NH_4NO_3
	Euglena gracilis	0.60	light, CO_2, NH_4
	(Pringsheim) *	0.25	dark, butyrate, NH_4
	Euglena gracilis var.	0.42	light, CO_2, NH_4
	bacillaris	0.42	dark, butyrate, NH_4
		0.48	light, medium Table 2
		0.34	dark, medium Table 2
Mammalian cells (in culture)	*Hela cells* (strain of human epithelium) †	0.34	See (118)

* Data from Myers (95).
† Data from Puck *et al.* (118).
All growth measurements carried out at the optimum temperature 23 to 30°C. A k value of 0.30 corresponds to a generation time ~1 day. It is to be noted that the growth rate of *E. coli* is ~61 times that of *E. gracilis*.

trient. Stirring or additional aeration was seldom used. Growth is estimated, as already indicated, by taking a reading of the optical density in a spectrophotometer at 750 mμ, or by cell counts in a Levy blood counting chamber. Although there is considerable variation in length and diameter, individual organisms were measured by using a calibrated eyepiece micrometer. The cultures in light became a very deep green, yielding 8 to 10 g (wet-weight) of organisms per liter of nutrient fluid after 7 days' growth. Yields from dark-grown cultures were less and the packed centrifuged organisms were a creamy white. Growth-rate curves for light-grown and dark-grown *Euglena* show the change in optical density with time and the log of number of cells versus time during the log phase of growth. It will appear that the growth rate in the light is greater; but only under ideal conditions does the growth rate in the dark approximate that in the light (see Myers, 95). Comparative growth rates of *Euglena*, with other microorganisms, and a tissue culture of human Hela cells are indicated in Table 3. Although the growth rate of *Euglena* is of the same order as that of other algae, it would be considered slow compared with bacterial cultures.

2   STRUCTURE

". . . me thinks it seems very probable, that nature has in these passages, as well as in those of Animal bodies, very many appropriated Instruments and contrivances, whereby to bring her designs and end to pass, which 'tis not improbable, but that some diligent Observer, if help'd with better *Microscopes,* may in time detect." (Robert Hooke, *Micrographia,* p. 116, Royal Society London, 1665, taken from R. T. Gunther, *Early Science in Oxford,* Oxford University Press, Oxford, 1938.)

Electron Microscopy

More penetrating methods for the study of the ultrastructure of cells are being evolved in many laboratories; these methods should give us a better understanding of cellular structure. Light microscopy, especially polarizing, phase, and interference microscopy, can supply useful information about the structure of cells and their organelles. However, the electron microscope takes one to a higher order of resolution. Its average working resolution for biological material using newer techniques in tissue preparation is <30 Å $(1 \text{ Å} = 10^{-4} \mu)$; under ideal conditions, resolutions <10 Å may be obtainable. This resolution is sufficiently good to allow us to see molecules with weights of the order of 50,000.

To prepare cells for electron microscopy, they are usually fixed with a cellular poison containing a metal. (The process of fixing the cells is extremely complicated; few metals or poisons are good fixatives.) Such fixation increases the electron density, hence the contrast of the structure. The techniques for tissue fixation and preparation for electron microscopy have been described by Palade (102, 104) and in several recent texts (107, 150). The most successful fixative to date is 1 per cent osmium tetroxide (OsO_4) buffered at neutral or alkaline pH (7.0 to 8.5). Many microorganisms swell during or after fixation, but this can be partially prevented by increasing the tonicity of the fixative with sucrose (0.15 M). After dehydration, the fixed material is embedded in an acrylic resin (*n*-butyl methacrylate) or epoxide resin which, when polymerized, possesses the right hardness and ductility for thin-sectioning. Sections <0.05 μ in thickness are cut from the polymerized block on a microtome with the use of a glass knife. Sections of this thickness permit electron penetration and, therefore, the ability of seeing through the tissue section rather than viewing a shadow or replica of it in the electron microscope. With these techniques, the electron microscope enables us to see the actual molecular morphology underlying structure. This structural information (*e.g.,* for chloroplasts, mitochondria, and microsomes) can be integrated with the rapid advance of research in the biochemistry of tissue cells.

Structure of Euglena

By means of electron microscopy, some of the *fine structures* of *Euglena* are revealed. An active *Euglena* as observed in the light microscope and a schematic sketch of its structures was shown in the frontispiece. Electron micrographs of a cross-section of a *Euglena* (Fig. 6) and its structures (Fig. 7) are also shown. Much has been written about the structure of *Euglena,* particularly about differences separating species. The electron microscope, together with other analytical tools, should introduce a new precision regarding these structural concepts. As already indicated in this discussion, the general morphology of *Euglena* is that of a typical cell. It has, however, besides a cell membrane, a pellicle or exoskeleton, flagella (one large and one rudimentary), an eyespot (stigma), and chloroplasts, as well as mitochondria, nucleus, pigment granules, and other cytoplasmic organelles. These structures will be described briefly and illustrated here so that the gross structure of the organism can be grasped before taking up in detail the specific organelles and their relationship to photosynthesis, pigment synthesis, motor responses, and the effects of the environment on them (164, 169, 170).

Pellicle. So far, the cell membrane of *Euglena* has not been resolved by the electron microscope. Its pellicle or exoskeleton is a membranous structure so arranged and joined over its entire surface that it permits the organism to elongate and contract. The exoskeleton appears to

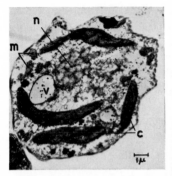

Fig. 6. Cross-section, electron micrograph (v, vacuole; c, chloroplast; n, nucleus; m, mitochondria).

Fig. 7. Electron micrographs. A. *Flagellum* (fixed in OsO_4 vapors, not sectioned) showing cilia-like mastigonemata and ring structure of flagellum sheath. B. Pellicle, note the ordered structure of the macromolecules that make up the organism's skeleton. C. *Gullet*, oblique section (fb, longitudinal fibrillae in the wall of the gullet; c_1, network of very fine fibrils; c_2, element of the endoplasmic reticulum; ap, ridges of the pellicle). D. *Mitochondria*, showing the cristae (or internal ridges) and the membrane. E. *Nucleus*, and large nucleolus with much granular material. F. *Chloroplast*, longitudinal section, to indicate its lamellar structure. G. *Eyespot*, system of 40 to 50 packed granules (orange-red).

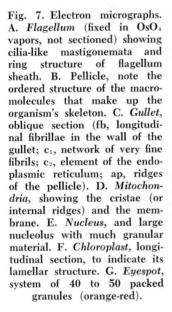

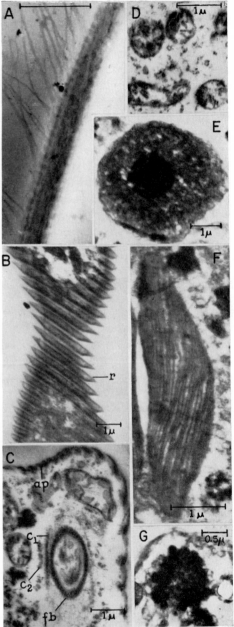

consist of a system of semi-rigid rings that alternate with strips of soft, pliable membrane. (Presumably, it is a non-cellulosic polymeric material; it would be extremely interesting to know its chemical composition.) It is seen in cross-section (Fig. 7B) to average from 0.1 to 0.25 μ in width. Examination of a large number of pictures of euglenas in various states of contraction gives the impression that the rings (or plates) slide into one another in the same manner as the abdominal rings of insects, or even as the rings of a collapsible cup (164, 169).

Chloroplasts. An active photosynthetic *Euglena* is bright green. The chloroplasts are sometimes referred to as *chromatophores* or *plastids* in *Euglena*. In different species and varieties, they vary in number from 1 to >20. They are elongated green bodies, more or less cylindrical in shape (Fig. 8), 1 to 2 μ in diameter, 5 to 10 μ in length, appear to have a limiting membrane, and contain, besides chlorophyll, carotenoids. Aside from their obvious relationship to photosynthesis, the chloroplasts are of considerable importance in the study of hereditary mechanisms.

Under the phase-contrast microscope, the chloroplasts show a faint lamination; in the polarizing microscope, they have both form and intrinsic birefringence. These observations pointed to an ordered structure below the limit of resolution of the light microscope. In fact, a "sub-microscopic" (by reference to the light microscope) structure had been postulated for chloroplasts in general on account of their birefringence. Some species of *Euglena* (*e.g.*, *E. spirogyra* and *E. granulata*) have huge chloroplasts that appear lamellar. These gross laminae are not comparable to those seen by electron microscopy.

Such an ordered structure was easily seen with the electron microscope (Figs. 6 and 7F). Fig. 6 shows at relatively low magnification a large area of a section through an active *Euglena* in which can be seen the profiles of four chloroplasts. A section through a single chloroplast is shown at a higher magnification, in Fig. 7F, where the elongated chloroplast is seen to be made up of a pile of discs or plates regularly spaced. Each disc is a continuous dense and homogeneous one of nearly uniform thickness. These discs in various electron micrographs are about 250 Å thick. From many electron micrographs, one gathers that the thickness varies according to the angle at which the section was cut, the thickness increasing as the angle of cut decreases. This would indicate that their thickness is probably closer to 200 Å. The interlamellar spaces vary from 300 to 500 Å and contain a less dense, almost colorless, homogeneous material, with very dense spherical granules embedded in it. The spacing

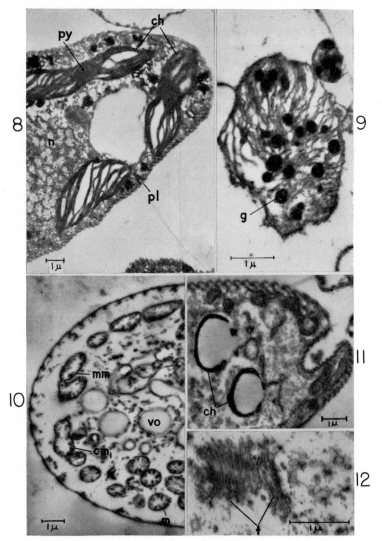

Fig. 8. *E. gracilis*, light-grown, longitudinal section indicating the profiles of the chloroplasts (ch), the pyrenoid (py), and the nucleus (n).
Fig. 9. Chloroplast, with its many dense granules (g), and the lamellae forming various patterns.
Fig. 10. *E. gracilis*, dark-grown, showing numerous *mitochondria*, with
limiting membrane (mm) and their cristae mitochondriales (cm), and
vacuole (vo).
Fig. 11. *E. gracilis*, dark-grown, with what appears to be collapsed
chloroplasts (ch).
Fig. 12. *E. gracilis*, dark-grown tubular elements (t) of the *endoplasmic reticulum.*

of the discs is affected by variations in fixation technique. At acid pH, for example, the lamellae seem to pull apart, often leaving large empty spaces between them.

The faint lamination shown occasionally by the chloroplasts of living euglenas under phase-contrast indicates some spacing irregularity in the living organisms. The lamellae themselves are too thin and closely packed to be resolved by light microscopy. Groups of lamellae separated by enough space may impart to the chloroplast the laminated appearance we have referred to. In the chloroplasts of inactive forms, the piling or stacking of the plates remains irregular whatever the precautions taken during fixation. In such euglenas, the plates seem distorted, and very frequently one finds them forming curious patterns in which they seem to converge in a central granule (Fig. 9). In such chloroplasts, the dense spherical bodies found between the lamellae are more numerous and more variable in size. When *Euglena* is dark-grown, the chloroplasts gradually fragment; their ultimate fate is unknown (Figs. 10 and 11). On being returned to light, *Euglena* again turns green, re-establishes its chloroplasts, and functions once more as a photosynthetic organism.

Pyrenoid. The pyrenoid is a differentiated region of the chloroplast. It is found in most green algae, but not in higher plants. It is an organelle concerned with starch synthesis and, in some algae, with lipid storage. In the elongated chloroplasts of active *Euglena,* one frequently finds a dense central region in which the lamellae seem to be held tightly together. In some preparations, their exact position, vis-à-vis the lamellae, can be ascertained, but in others, all trace of lamination disappears from this central region, and the pyrenoid is continuous as a condensation of interlamellar material. In some of our electron micrographs, the pyrenoid often protrudes at the surface of the chloroplast, the protrusion being frequently surrounded by a large cytoplasmic vacuole.

Mitochondria. The presence of mitochondria in *Euglena* and their general structure has been studied by Pringsheim and Hovasse (114). Palade and many others at the Rockefeller Institute have contributed much to knowledge of the structure and function of mitochondria (101). We find *Euglena* mitochondria not particularly different structurally from the mitochondria of protists, plants, and mammalian cells. In the electron micrographs, the mitochondria have two membranes: a limiting membrane 7 to 10 mμ thick and an inner membrane. A system of internal ridges protrudes from the inside surface of the inner membrane toward the interior. Generally, the ridges are perpendicular to the long axis of the mitochondria, but do not extend across the whole organelle. The ridges have been designated by Palade as *cristae mitochondriales* and consist of a series of cristae protruding from various sides (103). The mitochondria are seen in Figs. 7D and 10. It has been suggested that the oxidative enzymes of the mitochondria are built into these cristae. In the electron micrograph section of dark-adapted euglenas, the number of mitochondria is much increased; they are oriented toward the cell membrane and completely surround it (Fig. 10). In light-adapted organisms the distribution is less preferential, but the mitochondria surround the chloroplasts. Perhaps this means that the local oxygen tension, greater during photosynthesis, is a factor which helps determine the position of the mitochondria within the cell.

Endoplasmic Reticulum. This complex cytoplasmic system of vesicles and tubules was first revealed by the electron microscope in cultured animal cells. These structures have been described for practically all cells by Porter and Palade, who proposed that they correspond to the microsome fraction separated by differential centrifugation from tissue homogenates (105, 106, 112). The elements of this system may be integrated in a continuous network in the endoplasm. *Euglena,* like some animal cells, seems to have both bundles of tubular elements and a scattering of vesicular elements in its cytoplasm (Fig. 12).

Eyespot. The stigma or eyespot is believed to be the receptor for light perception. It is an orange-red body at the anterior end of the organism. As seen in the electron microscope, it is an agglomeration of numerous dense and randomly distributed granules. When packed together, there are 40 to 50 granules across its surface, each granule is $\sim$100 to 300 mμ in diameter. The cross-section of the whole eyespot in *E. gracilis* is $\sim$6 μ^2 (Fig. 7G); in *E. granulata* it is at least twice as large. The granules of the eyespot are located just below the membrane of the reservoir, a chamber with smooth walls that follows the ridged gullet from where the flagella originate. Between the granules and the membranes of the reservoir, one sees a system of regularly spaced fibrillae (Fig. 7C). Occasionally, a dense homogeneous body is seen attached to one of the flagella and facing the eyespot; it is denoted as the *paraflagellar body* (indicated by some as the photoreceptor).

Flagella. There are two flagella in *Euglena;* the importance of the second one is uncertain. It is considered that the elongated flagellum is the locomotor, whereas the rudimentary one is the rudder. The elongated flagellum is <30 μ long while the second is >5 μ. In some organisms, the second flagellum is missing. The flagella arise from two "roots" at the bottom of the gullet. In cross-section, the flagellum is 250 to 400 mμ in diameter. In sections, the flagella appear to consist of a number of elementary filaments (axonemata) embedded in a matrix and covered by a membrane. The elementary filaments number eleven pairs, of which nine are peripherally located while the other two are found in the center of the flagellum. This is the arrangement seen in a wide variety of plant and animal flagella (26, 27, 91, 108, 109). In addition, lash-like fibrils (mastigonemata) are around these flagella.

Nucleus. The nucleus is a large spherical body ~5 μ in diameter. The center of the nucleus is occupied by a large dense ovoid nucleolus. On treatment with fixatives, one or more dense bodies that resemble nucleoli are also seen in the nucleus. These structures have been referred to in the protozoological literature as caryosomes or endosomes (62, 63).

Euglena also contains vacuoles, starch granules (paramylum, not stainable with iodine) and other cytoplasmic particulates.

The relation of the structural to the functional aspects of the chloroplast as a light-trapping organelle for photosynthesis, and the eyespot as a light-trapping organelle for light searching, are discussed in Chapter 4; the flagellum plus eyespot as a photoreceptor system is discussed in Chapter 7.

3   PIGMENTS

"From the simplest substances, carbon dioxide, water, and sunlight, autotrophic plants produce enormous quantities of organic matter. . . . Synthesis of all this diverse vegetable material hinges upon photochemical reactions that take place within the green parts of plants." (H. H. Strain, *Ann. Rev. Biochem.* 13:591, 1944.)

General Characteristics

No attempt is made here to review comprehensively the chemistry of algal pigments, but some general characteristics will be described that will be helpful in following the discussion of the pigments in *Euglena*. The two main types of pigments found in the euglenoids are the *chlorophylls* and the *carotenoids*. The chemistry of the chlorophylls and the carotenoids is summarized by Rabinowitch (120); the carotenoids are more specifically discussed by Strain (143-146), Karrer (69), Goodwin (40–41), and Fox (32); the synthesis of porphyrins is described by Granick and Mauzerall (46-48, 93).

Chlorophylls. The green pigments, the chlorophylls, comprise the main photosynthetic pigment of the chloroplasts. They have a cyclic tetrapyrrolic structure with magnesium as their nuclei (at the center of the molecule). The chlorophyll molecule has the empirical formula $C_{55}H_{72}O_5N_4Mg$. The molecular structure, as shown in Fig. 13, has been described as tadpole-like in appearance, having a large "head"— the porphyrin part—and a long "tail"—the phytol part. The phytol ($C_{20}H_{39}OH$) is a long chain alcohol, containing a double bond, which is related to the carotenoids and can be regarded as derivable from vitamin A by hydrogenation. The chlorophylls are easily extractable

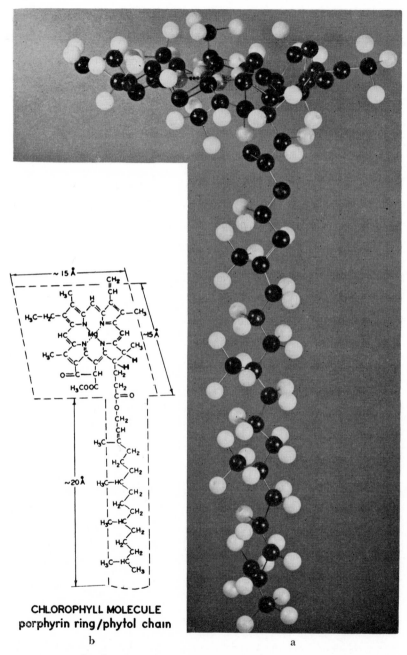

CHLOROPHYLL MOLECULE
porphyrin ring/phytol chain

b

a

Fig. 13. a. Molecular model for structure of chlorophyll. b. Structural formula of the chlorophyll molecule. Two hydrogen atoms, at positions 7 and 8 (in bold face), are added in the formation of chlorophyll from protochlorophyll.

from the cells in aqueous acetone or alcohol (80 to 90 per cent). The two higher plant chlorophyll isomers are: chlorophyll *a* and chlorophyll *b*. Chlorophyll *a* differs from chlorophyll *b* merely by the substitution of the methyl group at the 3-carbon, whereas in chlorophyll *b* a formyl (—CHO) group is in this position:

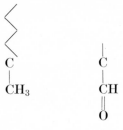

chlorophyll *a*   chlorophyll *b*

These chlorophylls differ in absorption spectra as shown in Fig. 14 for chlorophylls *a* and *b*, as well as in solubilities; *e.g.*, chlorophyll *a* is more soluble in petroleum ether while chlorophyll *b* is more soluble in methyl alcohol.

Pheophytin (*a* or *b*) is chlorophyll minus magnesium. This is ob-

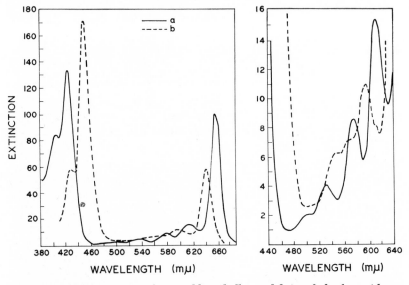

Fig. 14. Extinction curves of pure chlorophyll *a* and *b* in ethyl ether with an enlargement of the area between 440 and 640 mμ. ———— chlorophyll *a*; ------ chlorophyll *b* (after F. P. Zscheile and C. L. Comar, *Botan. Gaz.* 102: 463, 1941).

tained by treatment of the extracts with dilute acids. The conversion of chlorophyll into pheophytin can be followed spectrophotometrically by observing the gradual weakening of the red absorption band, accompanied by a change of color ("bleaching").

Seeds and etiolated plants (seedlings sprouted in darkness) are sometimes faintly green, although they contain no chlorophyll. Upon exposure to light, they turn green immediately. The substance responsible for this reaction is a chlorophyll precursor, *protochlorophyll*. It differs from chlorophyll in that it lacks two hydrogen atoms in positions 7 and 8, and is an oxidation product of chlorophyll *a*.

The biosynthesis of porphyrins and chlorophyll is illustrated schematically in Fig. 15 from Granick's studies of *Chlorella* (46, 47). The diagrammatic molecular structure of the first colored products, protoporphyrin 9 (which is pink) and magnesium protoporphyrin, are illustrated in Fig. 16.

Carotenoids. Carotenoids are found also in the chloroplasts, the eyespot, and in other cytoplasmic granules of *Euglena*. All photoreceptor systems, plant and animal, concerned with phototropism, phototaxis, and vision, have been shown to depend upon carotenoids or their derivatives for function. Carotenoids are easily and abundantly synthesized by plants; multicellular animals cannot synthesize them—they must obtain carotenoids by ingesting plants. Animals can then modify, even degrade, the molecule of the carotenoid pigments to serve their special needs. This ability seems an animal prerogative.

Carotenoids are yellow, orange, or red, fat-soluble pigments, widely distributed in animals and plants. Generically named for their most familiar representative substance, carotene, they are divided into two main groups: *carotenes* (hydrocarbons) and *xanthophylls* (oxygen-containing derivatives). The oxygen atoms can be in hydroxyl, epoxide, carboxyl, or methoxyl groups. From the structure elucidated by Karrer (69), they can be considered, at least theoretically, to be built up from isoprene units. The linear portion of the molecule is constituted of four isoprene (2-methyl-1,3-butadiene) residues. The isoprene units are linked so that the two methyl groups nearest the center of the molecule are in positions 1:6, while all other lateral methyl groups are in position 1:5. In chemical structure, the carotenoid molecule is made up of a chromophoric system of alternate single and double interatomic linkages, so-called conjugated double bonds, between the carbon atoms of a long chain. This is illustrated in Fig. 17; the absorption spectrum for β-carotene is given in Fig. 18.

Less is known of the manner of biosynthesis of carotenoids, but it

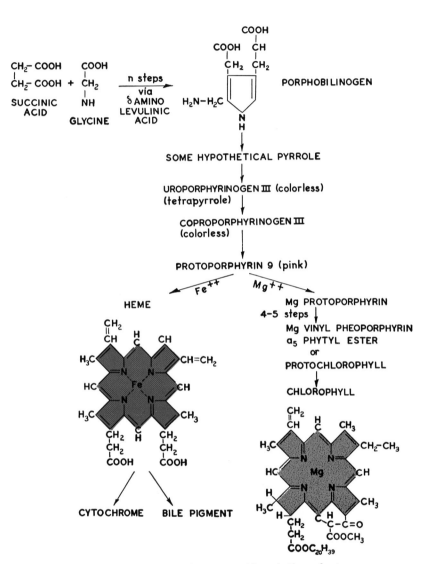

Fig. 15. Granick's scheme for chlorophyll synthesis.

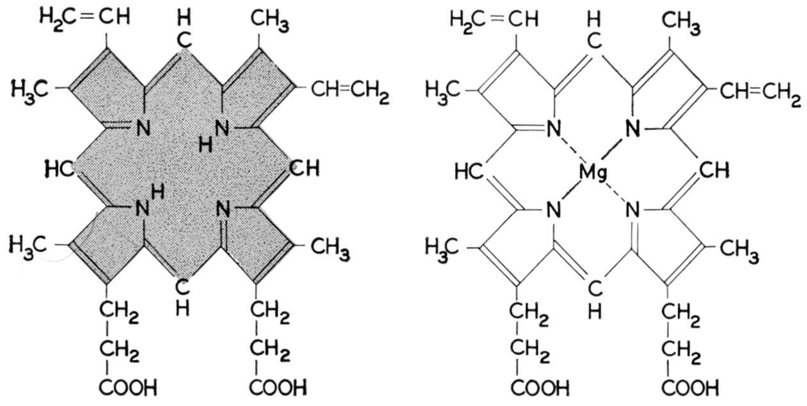

Protoporphyrin-9 Magnesium protoporphyrin-9

Fig. 16. Molecular formulae for protoporphyrin 9 and magnesium protoporphyrin.

is known that they are genetically associated with the 20-carbon atom aliphatic alcohol phytol, which is the colorless moiety of the ester comprising chlorophyll. The striking resemblance between the carotenoid skeleton and phytol holds also for the details of spacial configuration, which is similar to that which characterizes the carotenoids (see Fig. 19).

Pigment Analysis of Euglena

It would be very informative if the pigment synthesis in *Euglena* from light ↔ dark could be studied spectrophotometrically in a single organism, or better still, in the organelles, such as the chloroplast and the eyespot. Microspectrophotometric techniques, making this possible, are being developed in several research laboratories (147).

To obtain the absorption spectra (for identification of pigments), either the absorption spectra of a mass population of microorganisms is measured in a spectrophotometer or the pigments are extracted in appropriate solvents and further purified before their absorption spectra are determined. Obtaining absorption spectra of *Euglena* pigments *in vivo* is difficult, even in media, such as bovine albumin, which tend to correct for refractive index. The light-scattering difficulty can be circumvented to some extent by placing an opalescent material between the suspension of organisms and the photocell (130). The absorption peaks obtained in this way were at 675, 625, 590, and 485-

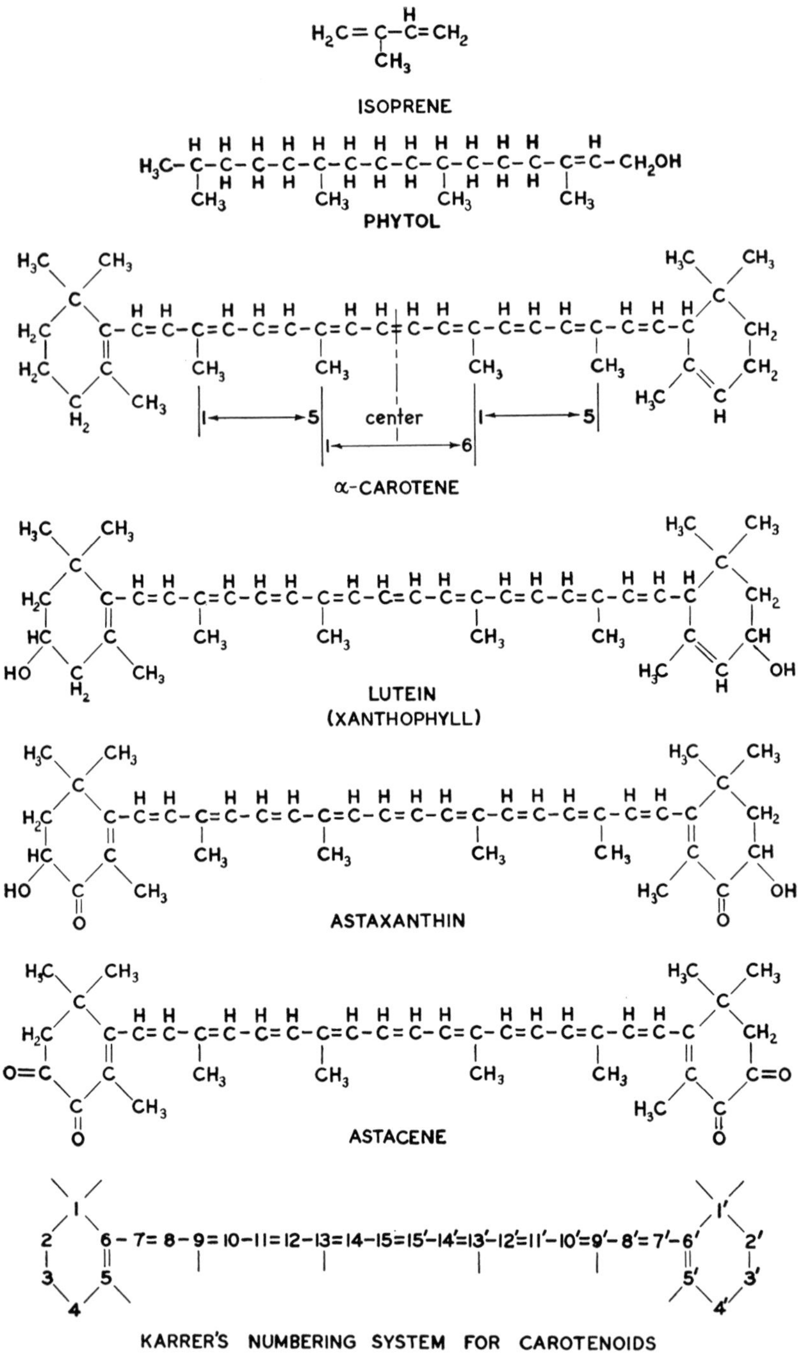

$$H_2C = \overset{\overset{\displaystyle H}{|}}{\underset{\underset{\displaystyle CH_3}{|}}{C}} - \overset{\displaystyle H}{C} = CH_2$$

ISOPRENE

$$H_3C - \overset{\overset{H}{|}}{\underset{\underset{CH_3}{|}}{C}} - \overset{\overset{H}{|}}{\underset{\underset{H}{|}}{C}} - \overset{\overset{H}{|}}{\underset{\underset{H}{|}}{C}} - \overset{\overset{H}{|}}{\underset{\underset{CH_3}{|}}{C}} - \overset{\overset{H}{|}}{\underset{\underset{H}{|}}{C}} - \overset{\overset{H}{|}}{\underset{\underset{H}{|}}{C}} - \overset{\overset{H}{|}}{\underset{\underset{CH_3}{|}}{C}} - \overset{\overset{H}{|}}{\underset{\underset{H}{|}}{C}} - \overset{\overset{H}{|}}{\underset{\underset{H}{|}}{C}} - \overset{\overset{H}{|}}{\underset{\underset{CH_3}{|}}{C}} = C - CH_2OH$$

PHYTOL

α-CAROTENE

LUTEIN
(XANTHOPHYLL)

ASTAXANTHIN

ASTACENE

$$2 \quad 6-7=8-9=10-11=12-13=14-15=15'-14'=13'-12'=11'-10'=9'-8'=7'-6' \quad 2'$$
$$3 \qquad 5 \qquad \qquad \qquad \qquad \qquad \qquad \qquad \qquad \qquad \qquad 5' \quad 3'$$
$$4 \qquad \qquad \qquad \qquad \qquad \qquad \qquad \qquad \qquad \qquad \qquad \qquad 4'$$

KARRER'S NUMBERING SYSTEM FOR CAROTENOIDS

Fig. 17. Molecular diagrams of carotenoid molecules.

30

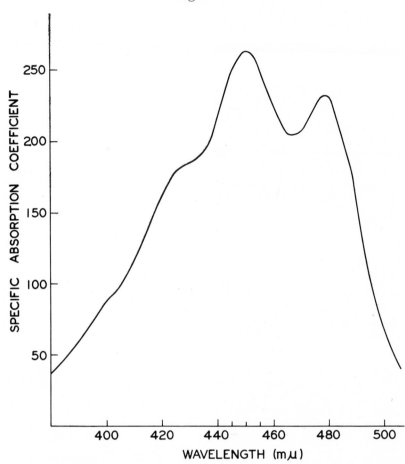

Fig. 18. Absorption spectrum of β-carotene in hexane (after F. P. Zscheile, T. W. White, B. W. Beadle, and J. K. Roach, *Plant Physiol.* 17:331, 1942).

488 mμ, and slight shoulders were found at about 460 and 437 mμ. This compares very well with digitonin extracts of *Euglena,* which have peaks at 675, 625, 590, and 488 mμ, and shoulders at 460, 437, and 417-421 mμ. This is indicated by the absorption spectra of a suspension of *E. gracilis,* compared to an aqueous digitonin extract (Fig. 20). The latter peak may be caused by pheophytin in the extract, which is probably present in the living cells.

After the pigments were extracted in solvents (methyl alcohol or acetone), the chlorophyll concentration was determined according to the method of Arnon (2), in which the concentrations of chlorophyll

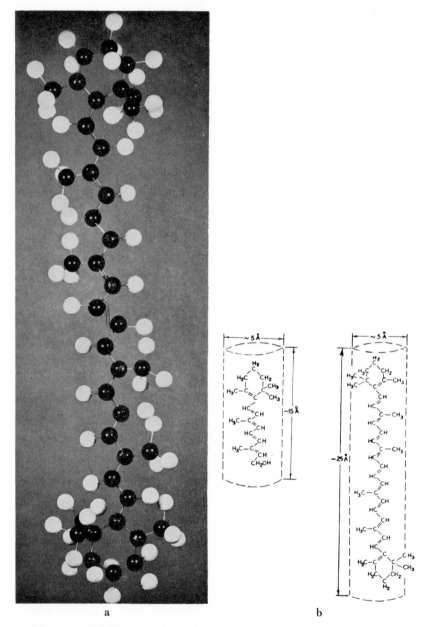

Fig. 19. a. Model for molecular structure of carotenoid molecule, β-carotene (in which two C_{20} units are joined together). b. Structural formula of vitamin A_1, the C_{20} unit (left), and the formula of β-carotene, the C_{40} unit (right).

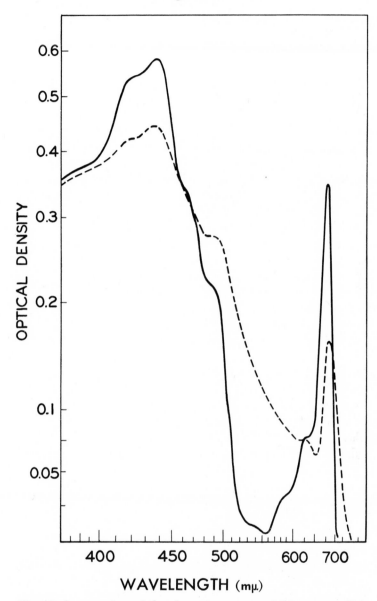

Fig. 20. A comparison of the absorption spectra of 1.8 per cent digitonin extract of a chloroplast fraction, and a suspension of *E. gracilis*. Recordings were made with Beckman DK recording spectrophotometer. ——— Chloroplastin, digitonin complex; ----- *in vivo E. gracilis*.

a and *b* are determined by measuring the optical density of the acetone-extracts at 663 and 645 mμ, using the specific absorption coefficients for chlorophylls *a* and *b* given by McKinney (88).

Attempts have been made to isolate both Mg vinyl pheoporphyrin and its phytol ester, protochlorophyll—the precursors in the biosynthesis of chlorophyll—from dark-adapted euglenas. Granick's method (46) was followed with the former, and Koski and Smith's (71) for protochlorophyll. Several porphyrin-like compounds were extractable from dark-adapted cultures. However, the only compound which has been tentatively identified from absorption spectra is protoporphyrin 9 (diagrammatic structure minus the phytol is illustrated in Fig. 16; see its place in Granick's scheme for chlorophyll synthesis). This porphyrin was found in *E. gracilis* which had been dark-grown for two weeks. The organisms were grown in 4-liter cotton-stoppered flasks containing 2 liters of medium. The cultures were stirred by bubbling clean, compressed, filtered air through them. The packed cells were pinkish-yellow. The cells were extracted in absolute alcohol, and then in 3:1 ethyl ether-absolute alcohol to remove fat-soluble pigments. The pellet was then stirred with 99:1 acetic acid-HCl (1 ml 6 N HCl), centrifuged, and extracted twice more. The extracts were combined and treated with 2 N potassium acetate to convert the pigments to a neutral form, and then extracted with ethyl ether. Protochlorophyll has recently been identified in dark-grown cultures of *E. gracilis* (98).

It is generally assumed that the pigment in the eyespot of *Euglena* is *astaxanthin,* mainly because of the discovery of astaxanthin in the cytoplasm of the red *Euglena sanguinea*. The pigment astaxanthin (α-hydroxydiketo derivative of β-carotene) has been encountered thus far only in animal tissue, in the eyes and in the integument of crustaceans (it is familiar as the red pigment of the boiled lobster), and occurs as a screening pigment in the retina of avians. The analysis by Tischer of the red pigment, haematochrome, from *E. heliorubescens* and from *Haematococcus pluvialis*, demonstrated that the principle component is euglenarhodon ($C_{40}H_{48}O_4$), a ketonic xanthophyll. This is also believed to be the pigment of *E. rubra* (67). This pigment resembles, or is believed to be identical with, astacene, a ketonic carotenoid thought to be a degradation product of astaxanthin isolated from crustaceans (153).

Evidence is lacking for participation of astaxanthin in the rhodopsin (visual-purple) cycle of the mammalian retina or in the metabolism of vitamin A. However, astaxanthin may act as the screening pigment for the photoreceptor. Identification of astaxanthin in plants would be most interesting. The absorption spectrum of crustacean astaxanthin, unlike those of the common plant carotenoids, is a single broad band, maximal in the blue-green. If the *Euglena* pigment is indeed astaxanthin, it would nicely befit the peculiar position in biology of the green flagellates—they alone would have both the plant pigment chlorophyll and the animal pigment astaxanthin. Unfortunately, neither we nor Goodwin and Jamikorn (43) have been able to detect astaxanthin in cultures of *E. gracilis*, even in the presence of streptomycin which bleaches almost all the chloroplast pigments, although the orange-red eyespot is still observable. In old cultures of the *E. gracilis* Z strain, the eyespot granules became quite large and scattered randomly throughout the cell. An orange-red fraction could be isolated after grinding the cells by differential centrifugation. This fraction dissolved in saline had an absorption spectrum with a broad peak between 420 and 440 mμ and a shoulder between 470 and 480 mμ, indicative of β-carotene.

The failure to observe astaxanthin may be that it is present only in traces; on the other hand, the bright orange-red color of the eyespot area indicates the presence of a concentrated pigment. Astaxanthin has only one absorption peak, not sharp, with a maximum density at 500 mμ sloping off to half that density at 460 and 560 mμ (40). The presence of chlorophyll is not responsible for our failure to find astaxanthin, as the absorption of chlorophyll is low at 480 to 500 mμ. Also, as noted, streptomycin treatment reduces both the chlorophyll and carotenoid concentration, still leaving the eyespot pigment. We have no data on the specific absorption of astaxanthin, only on its relative extinction coefficients from 400 to 600 mμ. Such an absorption peak would be given by any pigment showing sharper curves; the pheophytin absorption peak at 505 mμ would completely mask it.

Extracts of dark-grown organisms indicate that two carotenoids which persist in the dark are lutein and β-carotene. These are two of the carotenoids identified (Table 4) by Goodwin and Jamikorn (43) in dark-brown euglenas.

Chromatography of Pigments. The separation of the *Euglena* pigments on adsorption columns by chromatographic methods has been carried out. The adsorption columns used were $\frac{2}{3}$ sucrose, $\frac{1}{6}$ CaCO$_3$, and $\frac{1}{6}$ special chromatographic alumina. The pigments were adsorbed from a 9:1 benzene-petroleum ether (bp 34.5-55°C) solution. In most

TABLE 4

Separation of the Carotenoids of *E. gracilis* (43)

Zone no.	Descrip-tion	Spectral absorption maxima in light petroleum (in mμ)	Identifi-cation
I	brown-khaki	~422, 448, 475	β-carotene
II	lemon-yellow	~419, 442, 469	lutein
III	yellow	415, 438, 463	neoxanthin

Adsorbent: weakened alumina; developer: light petroleum ether containing different amounts of diethylether. ~ Denotes an inflection.

cases, the pigments separated on this column; two green bands were observed on the sucrose, several yellow bands on the $CaCO_3$, and an orange band on the alumina. Distinct peaks for chlorophyll *a* and chlorophyll *b* were obtained. The best data for determining chlorophylls *a* and *b* on samples which showed little evidence for the presence of pheophytin indicated that chlorophyll *b* ranged from 15 to 20 per cent of the total amount of chlorophyll. In *E. gracilis* cultures from 2 to 15 days old, chlorophyll *b* averaged 13.3 per cent; the percentage decreased with age of the culture. The chlorophyll distribution in *E. gracilis* can therefore be considered as 85 per cent chlorophyll *a* and 15 per cent chlorophyll *b*.

The pigments were also chromatographed on Whatman No. 1 filter paper. This gave three spots when the extraction was done quickly in a very dim green light and chromatographed in the dark with appropriate solvents. The pigments were originally extracted in 85 per cent acetone and shaken with a small amount of petroleum ether in a separatory funnel. The petroleum ether was washed with water to remove the acetone, and discarded, leaving the pigments in the petroleum ether. This was applied to one corner of a square of filter paper, previously washed with a mixture of petroleum ether, methanol, and acetone, in equal proportions, and chromatographed in the first dimension with benzene and in the second dimension with petroleum ether in an atmosphere of methanol. The three pigments isolated in this way were chlorophyll *a*, chlorophyll *b*, and β-carotene. Their absorption peaks in 85 per cent acetone are indicated in Table 5. A yellow pig-

TABLE 5

SEPARATION OF CAROTENOIDS BY PAPER CHROMATOGRAPHY

Pigment	Absorption peaks in mµ
Chlorophyll *a*	662, 618, 575, 532, 430, and pheophytin at 410-412
Chlorophyll *b*	648 and 460
Carotenoids	
β-carotene	430, 451, and 479
lutein and/or neoxanthin	412, 439, and 466

ment (probably lutein, neoxanthin, or both) which appeared on many of the chromatograms had absorption peaks in 85 per cent acetone around 412, 439, and 466 mµ, in agreement with Goodwin's data (Table 4). Recent attempts by Krinsky and Goldsmith (72) have been made to identify the carotenoids by chromatography of *E. gracilis* eyespots. They also were unable to detect either astaxanthin or astacene. However, they did find β-carotene, γ-carotene, echinenone, and cryptoxanthin.

The relative amounts of carotenoids found in two different varieties of *E. gracilis* by Goodwin and Jamikorn (43) and in bleached substrains of *E. gracilis* (42) are tabulated in Table 6.

TABLE 6

PERCENTAGE AMOUNTS OF THE COMPONENT CAROTENOIDS IN TWO VARIETIES OF *E. gracilis*

Pigment	v. *bacillaris* *	v. *fuscopunctata* †
β-carotene	11	15
lutein	82	16
neoxanthin	7	21

* Seven days growth.
† Age of culture unknown.

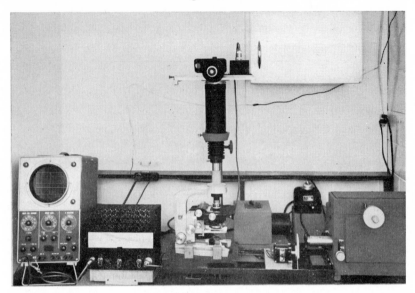

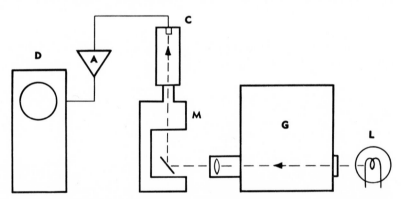

Fig. 21. Photograph and diagram of microspectrophotometer. L, light source; G, monochromator; M, microscope with reflecting optics; C, photoconductive cell; A, amplifier; D, oscilloscope.

Microspectrophotometry. To study the pigments and pigment changes in the chloroplast and the eyespot, a microspectrophotometer (shown in Fig. 21) was designed and constructed using reflecting optics in the light microscope with a cadmium selenide photoconductive cell as the light-sensitive element (147). Light from source L enters a grating monochromator G. The exit slit of the monochromator is focused by a quartz lens on the condenser of the microscope, M. After passing through the specimen, the light beam hits the photo-sensitive cell C, accurately positioned above the microscope eyepiece. The electrical signal from the photocell is amplified by A, a transistorized dc amplifier, and displayed on D, a Dumont oscilloscope.

Absorption spectra of cell suspensions do not permit spectra from the individual organelles, and therefore *fine structure* details are not obtainable. Spectra can easily be obtained by using the microspectrophotometer for the *in vivo* chloroplast and eyespot of *Euglena*. The absorption spectra in Fig. 22 are from individual chloroplasts and extend over a wavelength range of 250-700 mμ. Except for changes in relative peak heights, consistent data can be obtained providing the conditions of growth are kept constant. This permits then a study

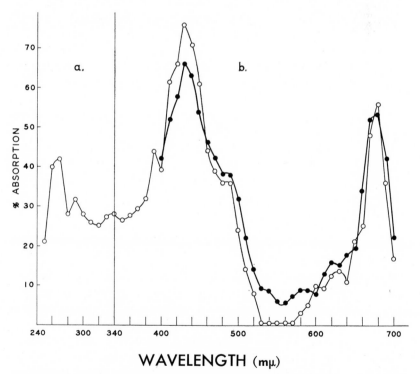

Fig. 22. *E. gracilis* chloroplast absorption spectra. a. Ultra-violet absorption over the range 250 to 340 mμ. b. Visible absorption over the range 340 to 700 mμ of two different chloroplasts.

of the chloroplast pigments with changes in the environmental conditions (nutrition, time, light intensity).

The absorption peaks in the region of 265-270 mμ and minor peaks at 290, 340, and 390 mμ are probably due to the proteins and lipids in the chloroplast. In the visible spectrum, these chloroplasts have two major absorption peaks, one in the region 430-435 mμ and the other in the region 675-680 mμ, with minor peaks near 485, 585, and 620 mμ. The 485 mμ is known to be a carotenoid; the other absorption peaks, in Fig. 22b, are mainly due to chlorophyll *a*. As the culture ages, changes occur in the 415-435 mμ and new peaks in the region of 680-695 mμ were observed (147a, 165a).

The eyespots were investigated in the visible range, 400-700 mμ. The reference area was the cell cytoplasm or the vacuole adjacent to the eyespot. The spectrum for an average eyespot is illustrated in Fig. 23. In contrast to the chloroplast spectra, the eyespot data exhibited appreciable variation in peak height from one eyespot to another. The data show that the eyespot has a broad absorption maximum in the region 480-490 mμ, two sharper maxima at 510 and 530 mμ, and lesser peaks at 430 and 630 mμ. The eyespot therefore absorbs light throughout the entire visible range. The action spectrum for *Euglena* phototaxis has peaks at 420 and 490 mμ. For photokinesis (rate of swimming irrespective of direction), *Euglena* has peaks at 465 and 630 mμ. An absorption peak at 450-460 mμ was noted for several eyespots, and is shown as a shoulder on the curve in Fig. 23. This spectrum is in agreement with that obtained by Gössel using a microbeam larger than the eyespot cross-section (44). It is also of interest to compare the eyespot absorption spectrum of *E. granulata*, whose eyespot is much larger and appears more red than orange in color (165b, c). The eyespot absorption spectrum of *E. granulata* has absorption peaks at 410, 460, 510, and 540 mμ; many of these same absorption peaks are found for the eyespot spectrum of *E. gracilis* (Fig. 23).

Pigmented structures resembling eyespots are found within euglenas of old cultures. These "hematochrome flecks" appear in various parts of the cell, and a single organism could have as many as five (60). Their most characteristic color was brown to dark red, and grana were clearly evident within them. Because of their similarity to the eyespots, absorption spectra were obtained. As might be expected from their appearance, they exhibited general non-specific absorption throughout the entire visible range. However, absorption peaks near 425, 460, and 480 to 490 mμ were consistently found in all the euglenas investi-

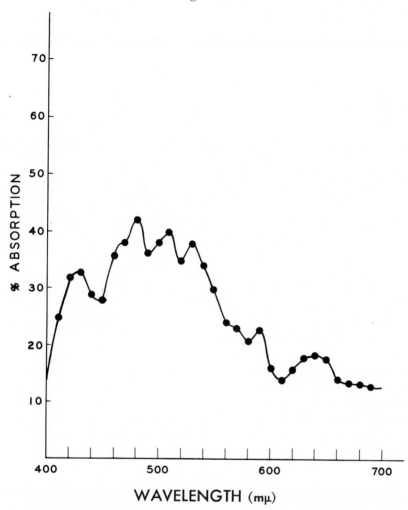

Fig. 23. *E. gracilis* eyespot average absorption spectrum.

gated. Since these same peaks are in the eyespot spectra, the "hema-tochrome flecks" may be eyespots which have undergone an increase in number and in size and have migrated throughout the cytoplasm. The interpretation of Fig. 23 with respect to the identity of the pigments present in the eyespot is, however, difficult. *E. gracilis* pro-duces three main carotenoids: β-carotene, lutein, and neoxanthin. The absorption range of these carotenoids is from 450-510 mμ and could, therefore, account for the observed absorption.

4   PHOTORECEPTORS

"Nowhere do mathematics, natural science, and philosophy permeate one another so intimately as in the problem of space." (H. Weyl, *Philosophy of Mathematics and Natural Science*, p. 67, Princeton University Press, 1949.)

Photoreceptors are organelles of living cells containing photosensitive pigments that upon light absorption initiate phototropisms, photosynthesis, and vision. *Euglena* has two photoreceptors, the *chloroplast* and the *eyespot*. The eyespot is the organism's receptor for light-searching, directing *Euglena* by phototropic reactions to light for chlorophyll absorption within the chloroplast, thus enabling *Euglena* to carry on photosynthesis. In the alga *Chlamydomonas*, the eyespot and the chloroplast are associated together within the chloroplast membrane (124), suggesting that there must be a functional relationship between these two photoreceptors.

The Chloroplast

The site of photosynthesis in plant cells is the chloroplast. Its chemistry and structural organization must therefore be intimately linked with photosynthesis. Because of this, it is necessary to know the molecular structure of the chloroplast if we are to understand how it functions in energy storage and transfer.

Euglena is ideally suited for the study of the chloroplast structure since, as previously described, it is photosynthetic in the light and "chemosynthetic" in the dark. These light ↔ dark adaptations are accompanied by biochemical and structural changes of the organism

42

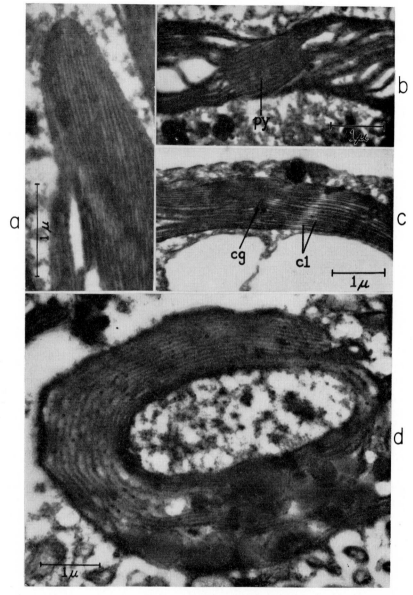

Fig. 24. Electron micrographs of sectioned chloroplasts in *Euglena*, *py* indicates pyrenoid; *cg*, chloroplast dense granules; *cl*, chloroplast lamellae. *a*, *b*, and *c* are *E. gracilis*; *d* is *E. granulata*.

and particularly the chloroplast. Evidence from electron microscopy, for a variety of plants, shows that the active chloroplast consists of piled-up plates or discs described as lamellae (Fig. 24). When taken from the light and grown in the dark, *Euglena* disrupt their chloroplast lamellae and with continued growth in the dark the chloroplasts become no longer recognizable. To find out what happens to the chloroplasts on dark-adaptation of *Euglena*, Pringsheim *et al.* (114, 115) tried to follow these changes by conventional microscopic methods. It is now possible to study more precisely the chloroplast disruption and development with the electron microscope. The dark-grown euglenas, whose chloroplast structures were no longer recognizable, were brought back into the light, fixed at regular time intervals, and the structural formation of their chloroplasts followed by electron microscopy. It was found that, after as little as four hours in the light, elongated bodies with the characteristic lamination of the chloroplasts began to appear. With continuous light, the lamellae, few in number at first, increased progressively with time, but these lamellae were thinner and not regularly packed; after 72 hours light, the chloroplasts had the shape and structural organization described for active euglenas grown in light for generations. What has thus far been seen in dark-grown *Euglena* exposed to light does not permit any definite conclusions concerning the origin and development of new chloroplasts (166). However, the formation of lamellae is dependent on chlorophyll synthesis (164, 165, 166a).

Geometry. Let us then explore the spacial arrangement (geometry) of the actively photosynthesizing chloroplast by microscopy and electron microscopy to see whether this data would provide us with information for a molecular structure of the chloroplast.

From a population of *E. gracilis* (more than 100 organisms), the number of chloroplasts and their outer dimensions (diameter and length) were measured and averaged (Table 7). The microspectrophotometer was then employed to scan across the *in vivo* chloroplast at the major absorption peak for chlorophyll (675 mμ) at 0.5 μ intervals (Fig. 25). This revealed that its photosensitive pigment, chlorophyll, is evenly distributed throughout the whole chloroplast.

E. gracilis was then fixed for electron microscopy; the resolution was sufficiently good to clearly delineate dense layers (lamellae) and less dense interspaces (Fig. 24). The dense layers were counted and the thickness measured (Table 7). The chloroplasts were found to consist of an average of 21 layers of the order of 250 Å in thickness.

TABLE 7

CHLOROPLAST GEOMETRY IN *E. gracilis*

Symbol	Definition	Arithmetic mean
W (microns)	Diameter	1.23 (1.04-1.42) *
d (microns)	Length	6.5 (5.2-9.3)
n	Number of dense layers	21 (18-24)
T (Angstroms)	Dense layer (disc) thickness	242 (180-303)
I (Angstroms)	Interspace thickness	374 (300-476)

* Extreme values.

Each dense layer appears as a double layer whose denser surfaces (lamellae) are from 50 to 100 Å in thickness. The interspaces are more variable and range from 300 to 500 Å in thickness. There are at present no chemical analyses of these layers. The dense layers are considered lipids and lipoproteins, because of their affinity for osmium tetroxide used in fixation, and the clear spaces are thought to be aqueous proteins.

To see how much chlorophyll was available in the chloroplast volume and what area of the total surface would be occupied by the chlorophyll molecules, the chlorophyll concentration was determined. From suspensions of *E. gracilis*, during the log phase of growth, the pigments were acetone-extracted and the chlorophyll concentration calculated from spectroscopic data according to the method of Arnon (2). Knowing the number of moles of chlorophyll, the number of chlorophyll molecules per cell, C, was calculated from the equation:

$$C = \frac{m \times 6 \times 10^{23}}{E}$$

in which m is the calculated number of moles of chlorophyll, 6×10^{23} is Avogadro's number, and E is the number of organisms. Knowing

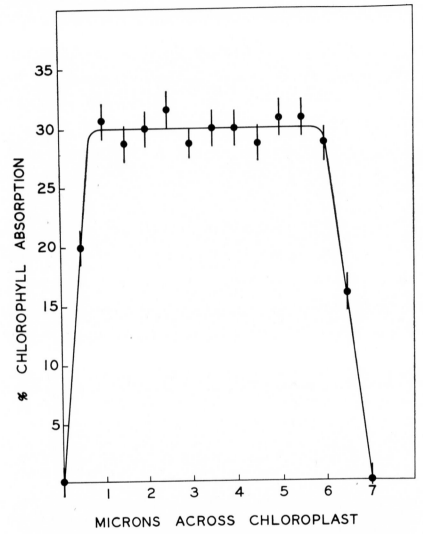

Fig. 25. The distribution of chlorophyll in the chloroplast, scanned across the chloroplast of *E. gracilis* with the microspectrophotometer (675 *vs.* 550 mμ).

C, and the average number of chloroplasts (p) per *Euglena*, the number of chlorophyll molecules (N) per chloroplast is easily obtained, *i.e.*, N = C/p. These results are summarized in Table 8.

Previously it was hypothesized that the chloroplast is a lamellar structure in which alternate parallel lipid layers are separated from

TABLE 8

CHLOROPHYLL CONCENTRATION IN *E. gracilis*

Symbol	Definition	Arithmetic mean
P	Average number of chloroplasts per cell	5 (4.0-7.0) *
C	Chlorophyll molecules per cell	5.1×10^9 (4.0-6.8)
N	Chlorophyll molecules per chloroplast	1.02×10^9 (0.88-1.36)

* Extreme values.

layers of aqueous protein by a film of chlorophyll molecules, the hydrophilic porphyrin "head" of each chlorophyll molecule extending into the aqueous protein, and the lipophilic phytol "tail" reaching into the lipid layer (35). The geometrical and analytical data taken together are consistent with such an ordered structure within the chloroplasts.

The validity for a monomolecular layer of chlorophyll molecules on the surface of the lamellae was then determined by calculating the area available for the porphyrin head of the chlorophyll molecule. The calculation is possible on the basis that the chloroplasts are disc-shaped and uniform in length. The longest chloroplast observed did not exceed the average length by more than 50 per cent, and very few chloroplasts measured less than one-half the average length.

These same observations apply when a knife is used to randomly slice through the face of a disc-shaped model. The average of a cut in this situation is $\pi/4$ times the diameter of the disc. Unless the flat surface of the knife were inclined toward the disc surface at an angle which was very different from 90°, the thickness of the cut would deviate little from the true thickness of the disc. For example, a cut at 45° to the disc surface is only about 40 per cent thicker than a 90° cut. The circular surface of this disc-shaped model has a cross-sectional area of $\pi D^2/4$. As shown above, $D = (4/\pi)d$, in which d is the average observed length of the chloroplasts. The cross-sectional area is therefore $(4/\pi)d^2$. When there are n lipid (dense) layers, there are $2n$ interfaces available to the chlorophyll molecules, and hence

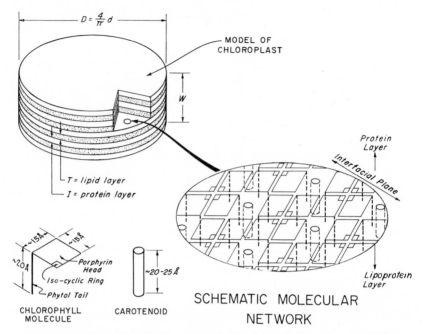

Fig. 26. Schematic molecular network for chlorophylls and carotenoids.

the total area of $(8/\pi)nd^2$. The area, A, accessible to each chlorophyll molecule is then given by:

$$A = \frac{(8/\pi)nd^2}{N}$$

in which N is the average number of chlorophyll molecules per chloroplast. By employing the values of these quantities presented in Tables 7 and 8, the available cross-sectional area obtained for A is 222 Å^2 for *E. gracilis*. If the same analysis is carried out for the chrysomonad *Poteriochromonas stipitata*, a cross-sectional area of 246 Å^2 for the chlorophyll molecule is obtained. Calculations since made for the chlorophyll cross-sectional area in the chloroplast are also of the order of 200 Å^2 in a variety of plants (22).

On the basis of these considerations, a schematic molecular model, illustrated in Fig. 26, was proposed (170), following the suggestion of Baas Becking and Hanson (4) that four chlorophyll molecules are united to form tetrads in which the reactive isocyclic rings turn toward each other in an enlarged area of the chloroplast lamellar monolayer. Interaction between the phytol tails is eliminated by arranging the tetrads in such a way that one, and only one, of the phytol tails is located at each intersection in the rectangular network. This arrangement has the advantage of leaving adequate space for the carotenoid pigments. If these spaces were occupied as illustrated, there would be at least one carotenoid molecule for every three chlorophyll molecules in the network. Since the molecular weights of the carotenoid molecules are one-half to two-thirds of the molecular weight of the chlorophyll molecules, a weight ratio, chlorophyll to carotenoid, of approximately 4:1 to 6:1 would be expected.

On the other hand, the carotenoid molecules are slender linear molecules, probably less than 7 Å in diameter, and therefore more than one molecule could conveniently fit into the 15 Å × 15 Å holes formed by the chlorophyll tetrads. From symmetry, one might expect as many as four molecules per hole, but this would lead to very tight fitting which would be energetically improbable. One can, therefore, put a lower limit on the number of chlorophyll to carotenoid molecules of roughly one to one and a weight ratio of two to one. These figures are consistent with available data given by Rabinowitch (120). Other chloroplast models, however, modified from the one presented here, indicate that the chlorophyll molecules may also be turned inward (55). Calvin (13) has presented a similar chloroplast model for

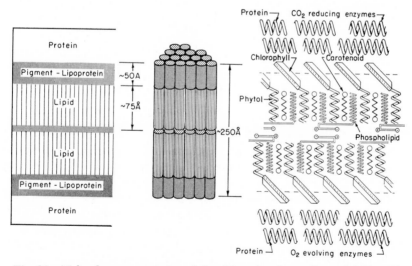

Fig. 26a. Molecular representation of the chloroplast layers (in model Fig. 26) showing orientation of chlorophyll molecules, CO_2-reducing and O_2-evolving enzymes in aqueous protein layers, from Calvin (13).

the orientation of the chlorophyll and carotenoid molecules, but in the alternate aqueous protein layers O_2-evolving and CO_2-reducing enzymes are included (Fig. 26a). The close packing of the chlorophyll and carotenoid molecules in the pigment monolayers, as depicted in these molecular models, would permit energetic interaction between the pigment molecules.

It is of interest to compare the chlorophyll concentration for the chloroplast of *E. gracilis* with that found for a higher plant, *Elodea densa*, and a moss, *Mnium* (Table 9). The average number of chloro-

TABLE 9

CHLOROPLAST VOLUME AND CHLOROPHYLL CONCENTRATION

Organism	Volume of chloroplast (in ml)	Chlorophyll molecules per chloroplast	Concentration of chlorophyll (moles per liter)
Elodea densa	2.8×10^{-11}	1.7×10^9	0.10 *
Mnium	4.1×10^{-11}	1.6×10^9	0.065 †
Euglena gracilis	6.6×10^{-11}	1.02×10^9	0.025
Poteriochromonas stipitata	1.1×10^{-11}	0.11×10^9	0.016

* Reference 155.
† Reference 37.

phyll molecules in the interfacial layers is obtained by simply dividing the chlorophyll concentration by twice the number of dense layers; hence the number would be 25×10^7 molecules per layer. The number of chlorophyll molecules per unit area in the interfacial monolayers is of course just the reciprocal of the area available to each molecule, *i.e.*, approximately 4×10^{13} per cm². Data for a variety of other plant chloroplasts have been obtained by Thomas (152) and indicate similar concentrations of chlorophyll to the chloroplast volume. The relative constancy of the number of chlorophyll molecules per chloroplast, and the volume of the chloroplast, suggest that chloroplasts possess a similar structural arrangement in a variety of photosynthetic microorganisms and higher plants.

The data on the fine structure of the chloroplasts and chlorophyll analysis are consistent with the hypothesis that the chlorophyll molecules are arranged in monomolecular layers at the interfaces between the lipid and the aqueous protein layers (35, 38). However, there are several possible ways in which the chlorophyll molecules could be oriented in the lamellae. If the porphyrin heads of the chlorophyll molecules lay at 0° as flat plates, as indicated in Figs. 26 and 27, their greatest cross-section would be available. However if they were oriented at increasing angles up to 90°, the cross-sectional area available would then be decreasing. Experimental studies of chlorophyll monolayers at various liquid surfaces suggest that the chlorophyll molecules would probably lie at an angle of 35 to 55° within the lamellae, thus reducing the cross-section of the chlorophyll molecule to about 100 Å². Chlorophyll *a* has been shown to crystallize out in thin sheets of 50 Å, corresponding to perhaps two-molecular layers. The crystallized chlorophyll molecules occupied an area of 106 Å² (61). The porphyrin part of the chlorophyll molecule is probably then tilted at an angle near 45°. The absorption oscillators of these pigment molecules are probably arranged in an orderly orientation in such a way that a maximum absorption will occur for an incident light polarized in a given direction.

Molecular Weight of the Chlorophyll Macromolecule. According to the chloroplast model (Fig. 26), there are monomolecular layers of pigments at the interfaces between the dense and less dense layers.

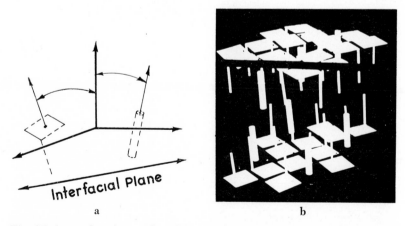

Fig. 27. Area taken from chloroplast model: a, the degrees of freedom of the chlorophyll and carotenoid molecules; b, the packing of the chlorophyll and carotenoid molecules at the interfacial planes.

The chlorophyll is not a free pigment molecule, but is complexed to a protein or lipoprotein macromolecule. The molecular weight of the chlorophyll macromolecule can then be calculated from the above data on the geometry and pigment concentration of the chloroplast.

On the assumption that the electron-dense layer would contain a double layer of macromolecules, the maximum cross-sectional area A, associated with each macromolecule and therefore with each pigment molecule, would be:

$$A = \frac{\pi D^2}{4P} \tag{1}$$

where D is the diameter of the photoreceptor and P is the number of pigment molecules in a single monomolecular layer. The *maximum* possible volume, V, associated with the macromolecule would then be:

$$V = \frac{\pi D^2 T}{8P} \tag{2}$$

where T is the average thickness of the double layer. The maximum chlorophyll macromolecule molecular weight M, would then be:

$$M = \frac{\pi D^2 TsL}{8P} \tag{3}$$

where s is the lipoprotein density and L is Avogadro's number. If N is the pigment concentration in molecules per chloroplast and n is the number of dense layers per photoreceptor,

$$P = \frac{N}{2n} \tag{4}$$

Equation 3 may therefore be written in a form containing only the experimental measurements:

$$M = \frac{\pi D^2 TsLn}{4N} \tag{5}$$

To calculate the molecular weight, M, the density for the protein, s, is taken as 1.3 g/cm^3. Using data for D, T, m, and N appearing in Tables 7 and 8, a calculated molecular weight of 21,000 was obtained.

The molecular weight can also be calculated from the *in vivo Euglena* chloroplast, using the Cook-Dyson Interference Microscope. This is done by obtaining the wave path difference of the chloroplast, and then calculating the molecular weight from the equation derived by Davies *et al.* (20):

$$M = \frac{\phi AL}{XP} \qquad (6)$$

($\phi = 1.1 \times 10^{-8}$ cm (for green filter λ 546 mμ) and 0.73×10^{-8} cm (for red filter λ 660 mμ); $X = 0.18$ constant; $A = 8 \times 10^{-8}$ cm^2, area of chloroplast; $P = 1 \times 10^9$ number of chlorophyll molecules per chloroplast; $L = 6 \times 10^{23}$) where M is the mass or the gram molecular weight associated with the chlorophyll-macromolecule, ϕ is the optical path difference, experimentally determined, of chloroplast, A is the area of the chloroplast, X is a constant associated with the medium, P is the average number of chlorophyll molecules per chloroplast, and L is Avogadro's number. Knowing the area of the chloroplast and its pigment concentration from the previous experiments, it was possible to calculate M. The experimental values substituted in the above equation resulted in an average molecular weight of 16,000; this is of the same order of magnitude as the molecular weight calculated from the molecular model (equation 5). Frey-Wyssling (35) considers, from electron microscopy, that the lamellae are made up of globular macromolecules, and estimates that these macromolecules are of the order of 65 Å in diameter. The macromolecule would then consist of 16 chlorophyll molecules oriented on its surface, and have a molecular weight of the order of 68,000.

The Pigment-Complex, Chloroplastin. Chloroplasts can be isolated from euglenas and other plant cells. The whole chloroplastic material from the chloroplasts can be extracted by surface active agents. Detergents in solution form colloid aggregates, micelles; such micellar bodies have a very strong attraction for a great many of the more complex dye molecules. Commercially available non-ionic and ionic surface agents were tried in extracting the pigment-complex from the chloroplasts. The non-ionic recrystallized detergents, Digitonin (a non-ionic detergent ($C_{55}H_{90}O_{29}$) a digitalis glycoside, D-58, Fisher Scientific Company) and Nacconal NRSF (a non-ionic detergent, alkyl aryl sulfonate, National Aniline Division, Allied Chemical and Dye Corporation) were found superior to all other surface active agents tested. These are nitrogen-free detergents and therefore do not interfere with subsequent protein analyses of the complex. The ionic detergents Alkonal B, glycocholate, and taurocholate were also good solubilizing agents; however, they do not preserve the spectral and photochemical properties of the chlorophyll-complex. For a discussion of the mode of action and the physical and chemical properties of detergents, refer to Putnam (119). Digitonin, because of its properties, opens the pigment-lipid-lipoprotein layers of the chloroplast and forms chloroplastin micelles. As already indicated, each digitonin micelle has a minimum molecular weight of 75,000 (or 75 molecules), and three such micelles are formed in solution with a molecular weight of 225,000. However, the chloroplastin micelle has a molecular weight of 290,000 and would contain 225-450 chlorophyll molecules, 50-100 carotenoid molecules, and one molecule of the enzyme cytochrome-552 plus lipid and protein to maintain the molecular configuration depicted in Figs. 27 and 28a. These micelles could then be considered the minimum functional photosynthetic unit, analogous to that of the chromatophores of photosynthetic bacteria.

The chloroplasts of *Euglena* were extracted in 1.8 per cent recrystallized digitonin, leaving a clear green solution containing chlorophyll, carotenoids, and protein (164, 165, 166a). This complex is referred to as chloroplastin. The physical and chemical properties of chloroplastin bear a resemblance to the *in vivo* chloroplasts (*e.g.*, its absorption spectrum (Figs. 20 and 22) and its ratio of pigment, lipid, and protein.

The analytical ultracentrifuge pattern in Fig. 28a shows that chloroplastin sediments as a single component, indicating a homogeneous complex; in Fig. 28b, it indicates that the protein, bovine albumin, does not complex with digitonin, and that the albumin and digitonin sediment as two separate entities.

From the chloroplastin it was possible to obtain the dried weight of the complex, the weight of the detergent, the chlorophyll concentration, and the nitrogen concentration. With these data, as well as from its sedimentation determined from analytical ultracentrifugation, the molecular weight of chloroplastin was calculated (164, 165). The average sedimentation constant, S_{20} (in Svedberg units), for digitonin was 7.1×10^{-13}, and for chloroplastin 13.5×10^{-13}.

The molecular weights were calculated from the equation:

$$M = \frac{RTS_{20}}{D_{20}(1 - p\overline{V}_{20})}$$

where R, the gas constant, is 8.32×10^7 dynes/cm, T the absolute temperature, S_{20} the experimentally determined sedimentation constant, D_{20} the diffusion constant, p the density, and $\overline{V}_{20}$ the partial specific volume. The value for the diffusion constant D_{20} was taken

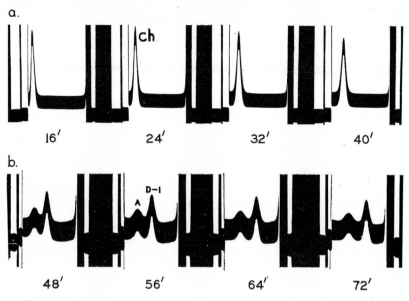

a.

ch

16'   24'   32'   40'

b.

D-1

A

48'   56'   64'   72'

a. 52,640 RPM
b. 56,100 RPM

Fig. 28. Analytical ultracentrifuge diagrams. (a) *Euglena* chloroplastin in digitonin; (b) Bovine albumin in digitonin.

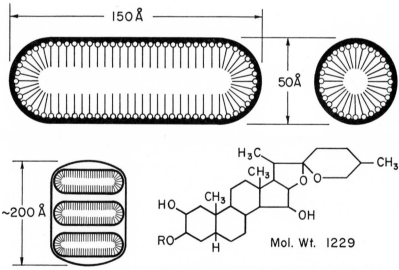

150 Å

50 Å

~200 Å

H_3C

CH_3 CH_3

CH_3

HO

RO

H

OH

O   O

Mol. Wt. 1229

R = 2 galactose + 2 glucose + 1 xylose

Fig. 28a. Digitonin structural formula. Purely schematic structure of digitonin micelle of about 75 molecules, and structure of three such micelles to form a large micelle of almost 225 molecules.

55

as 4×10^{-7} cm²/sec, and the partial specific volume $\overline{V}_{20}$ of 0.738 for the digitonin was obtained from Hubbard (57). Similar values for Nacconal, D = 10.3×10^{-7} cm²/sec, and $\overline{V}_{20} = 0.75$, were obtained from the data of Miller and Anderson (94). The calculated values are shown in Table 10. Nacconal forms micelles in water of a

TABLE 10

MOLECULAR WEIGHTS OF PIGMENT COMPLEXES
FROM ANALYTICAL ULTRACENTRIFUGE DATA

Chloroplast-complex	*Euglena gracilis* chloroplastin	*Poterio-chromonas* chloroplastin
1. Complex weight with digitonin	290,000	275,000
2. Complex weight with Nacconal	69,400	65,000
3. Molecular weight complex (minus digitonin micelle weight)	65,000	50,000
4. Molecular weight from Nacconal complex (minus Nacconal micelle weight)	31,900	27,500
5. Molecular weight from digitonin complex (minus digitonin * micelle weight)	57,500	42,500
6. Molecular weight from Nacconal complex (minus Nacconal † micelle weight)	31,150	26,750

* Experimental minimum digitonin micelle weight 155,000 (165).
† Experimental minimum Nacconal micelle weight 25,000 (94).

minimum molecular weight equal to 12,500 to 15,000, and Smith and Pickels (136) have shown that digitonin forms micelles of a minimum molecular weight equal to 75,000. Hubbard has demonstrated that three such micellar units of digitonin are probably associated together (57). Assuming a similar situation holds true for Nacconal, the results are shown in 1 and 2 of Table 10. From these values, the quantity $3 \times 75,000 = 225,000$ for the digitonin-complex weight and $3 \times 12,500 = 37,500$ for the Nacconal-complex weights have been subtracted to give the molecular weights indicated in 3 and 4. The molecular weights appearing in 5 and 6 of Table 10 were obtained by using three-halves of our experimental values for the detergent micelle weight (165).

From the analytical data for chloroplastin in Table 11, the molecular weight can also be calculated from:

$$M = \frac{w'(100)}{p(15)}$$

where M is the molecular weight of the pigment macromolecule, w' is the weight of nitrogen in milligrams associated with 1 ml of the extract, and p is the pigment concentration in moles per liter of extract. The calculated values of M are entered in Table 11. The other experimental data listed in Table 11 are M', the molecular weight

TABLE 11

Chloroplastin Extracted from *E. gracilis*

	"Digitonin" extract			"Nacconal" extract		
	1	2	3	1	2	3
w mg/ml	29.0	27.3	29.6	44.3	42.5	23.0
w' mg/ml	0.37	0.36	0.35	3.1	3.8	0.67
p moles/liter (calculated)	10×10^{-5}	9.4×10^{-5}	10.2×10^{-5}	6.4×10^{-4}	6.1×10^{-4}	3.6×10^{-4}
p' moles/liter (experimental)	4.2×10^{-5}	6.3×10^{-5}	7.7×10^{-5}	9×10^{-4}	9.0×10^{-4}	0.9×10^{-4}
M' g/mole (ultracentrifuge)	290,000	290,000	290,000	69,400	69,400	69,400
M calculated from M'	43,500	43,500	43,500	10,400	10,400	10,400
M calculated from nitrogen	59,000	38,000	30,000	23,000	28,000	50,000

of the complex as determined by the analytical ultracentrifuge, and w, the total dry weight in milligrams associated with 1 ml of the extract. The agreement between the values in Tables 10 and 11 is reasonably close, although the bases for the calculations are different.

From the chloroplastin data (Table 11), it is possible to show that one pigment molecule is associated with each protein molecule. This was done by demonstrating that the experimentally determined chlorophyll concentration, p, was substantially the same as p' calculated from the formula:

$$p' = \frac{w}{M'}$$

No recent experimental data are available for the molecular weight of algal chloroplastin for comparative purposes. The data for chloroplastin have previously been obtained from leaf extracts (spinach and *Aspidistra*), prepared and calculated, in a similar manner, from its sedimentation constant as determined by analytical ultracentrifugation. Smith (134, 135) and Smith and Pickels (136, 137) found molecular weights of the order of 265,000. This high estimate, compared to our values, is partly due to the contribution of the digitonin micelle. Takashima (148) crystallized a chlorophyll-lipoprotein complex (from an α-picoline leaf extract at low temperature), and from diffusion studies calculated its molecular weight to be 19,200. He also postulated that the pigment-complex would have two molecules of chlorophyll per lipoprotein macromolecule. Recently, Smith and Kupke (139) isolated from bean seedlings (*Phaseolus vulgaris*) a chlorophyll holochrome (in glycine-KOH, pH 9.6), and determined from its sedimentation constants (S_{20} 15.3 to 16.2) a molecular weight of 400,000. The number of chlorophyll molecules and the ratio of chlorophyll to protein in this complex were not known. Smith has since found that the molecular weight of the macromolecule is closer to the order of a million, and that there is one pigment molecule per protein molecule (138a).

These complexes cannot be considered pure compounds; the difference in molecular weight can come from protein impurities and/or from the fact that the proteins could be different in different plants.

To summarize: the molecular weight of the chlorophyll macromolecule has been calculated from the model, assuming that each chlorophyll molecule is bound to a single protein molecule. The contribution of the macromolecules to the total weight of the dried extract was then calculated from nitrogen analyses on the assumption that nitrogen comprised 15 per cent of the protein weight. A knowledge of this weight, together with the pigment concentration, permitted the calculation of the macromolecular weight. In addition, the molecular weight was determined by an independent method which *did not* involve the assumption that each pigment molecule was attached to one macromolecule. For this method, the analytical ultracentrifuge was used to determine the molecular weight of the pigment-complex, chloroplastin. The molecular weight was calculated on the assumption that the fractional weight of the protein macromolecule, in the complex, was the same as that in the dried extract. Here again, molecular weights were obtained which were in close agreement with values obtained by the previously described techniques. All of these calculated values are for the most part in agreement as to the order of magnitude (20,000 — 60,000) and are consistent with the proposed molecular model.

Periodicity and Crystallization. What we have observed from the chloroplast structure is suggestive of a crystalline or quasi-crystalline nature. I would like to discuss briefly, then, some experiments on the formation of periodic (lamellar) systems that resemble the chloroplast structure. Firstly, there is the Liesegang ring phenomenon, observed by Liesegang in the course of staining specimens for histological study by the Golgi technique (*i.e.*, the impregnation of potassium dichromate and silver nitrate into tissue). Liesegang's experiments are described by Hedges (52), and the theories are treated in a more recent review by Stern (142).

The formation of the ring structures can be observed if a drop of 15 per cent silver nitrate is placed on a sheet of gelatin, which has previously been impregnated with about 0.4 per cent potassium dichromate. The silver slowly diffuses into the gelatin, there reacts with the potassium dichromate, and silver dichromate is precipitated in the gelatin. Another example is that of gelatin saturated with ferric chloride; if a drop of potassium ferrocyanide solution is placed in the center, blue rings of ferriferrocyanide will be formed. The precipitation is not continuous, but forms a series of concentric rings separated by clear spaces in the gel. When molecules are in solution, they take up configurations of lowest energy. This leads to crystallization when the number of molecules in the solution exceeds a certain minimum value characteristic of those particular molecules. An example of such a periodic crystallization is that of salts crystallizing in colloids or proteins, *e.g.*, potassium dichromate in gelatin and sodium chloride in serum. The procedure is to place a drop of saturated potassium dichromate in gelatin solution on a microscope slide, evaporate it quickly, and transfer the slide to the microscope. It will be observed that crystallization begins around the periphery of the drop and proceeds by periods of rapid and slow growth. Light can modify these periodic structures if the reacting molecules are light-sensitive.

Now let us return to chloroplastin, the chlorophyll-complex in aqueous 1-2 per cent digitonin. Chloroplastin, when caused to flow through a capillary, becomes birefringent when observed through crossed polaroids; hence there is an alignment of the molecules in solution. If a drop of chloroplastin is evaporated rapidly from a surface, periodic structures will also be formed similar to those just described. When these chloroplastin structures are scanned with the microspectrophotometer at the major absorption peak for chlorophyll (675 mμ), chlorophyll is found within the rings (Fig. 29) and not in the inter-spaces (compare to electron micrographs of fixed chloroplasts, Fig. 24). These experiments indicate that, in chloroplastin, chlorophyll molecules become oriented in a crystal-like structure. This then sug-

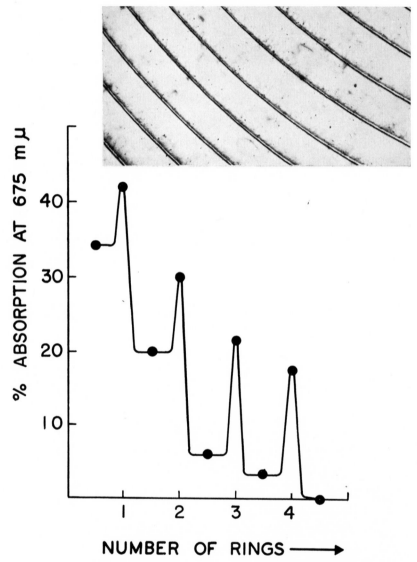

Fig. 29. Chlorophyll located in the ring structure of chloroplastin, as deter-mined with the microspectrophotometer.

gested a model system for study of photochemical reactions of the chloroplast in solution (see Chapter 6).

The question as to whether molecular structure tells us about chloroplast function as an energy storage and transferring device in photosynthesis has not as yet been completely answered. However, the experimental data suggest that the chloroplast is a kind of semiconductor—a photo-battery (1, 6).

The Eyespot

In the course of evolution, animals have developed various kinds of eye structures for light perception and image formation. The invertebrate, for example, developed sensory cells, ocelli, and compound eyes. The eyespot of *Euglena*, as the primary region for light reception and its analogy to the retinal cells of higher animals, was speculated as early as 1882 by Englemann (23). Further observations on *Euglena*, by Mast, indicated that a photosensitive pigment lay within the inner surfaces of the eyespot and not in front of it (92). Since the color of the eyespot (orange-red) implies absorption of light of the same wavelengths as are found to be effective in the phototropic reactions, the eyespot is indicated to be the photoreceptor. The eyespot and flagellum as a photoreceptor system of *Euglena* will be considered, together with the experimental studies on phototropic reactions, in Chapter 7. The eyespot contains carotenoids (see Chapter 3 and Fig. 23) not as yet specifically identified. These carotenoids are probably combined with lipids or proteins, but no such pigment-complexes have so far been isolated from euglenas.

The eyespot is about 2 μ in diameter and, in the electron microscope, is seen to consist of granules 100-300 mμ in diameter. There are 40-50 of these granules oriented at the base of the flagellum (see Figs. 30 and 31). When closely packed, they form a mosaic, suggesting that they are either rod or tube structures. It is to be noted that the eyespots appear structurally similar to the chromatophores of photosynthetic bacteria and blue-green algae. There are indications from electron microscopy of the eyespot granules' fine structure, that they too are lamellar structures, although it has been difficult to clearly resolve the lamellae. Between the eyespot granules and the membrane of the gullet, a system of regularly spaced fibrillae (a lamellar system) is found and is suggestive of the lamellar structure of most photoreceptors. Occasionally a dense homogeneous body attached to one of the flagella facing the eyespot is seen and lens-like structures are also

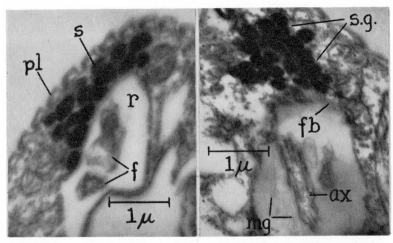

Fig. 30. Electron micrographs of the eyespot granules oriented near the base of the flagella in *E. gracilis*. pl, pellicle; s and s.g., eyespot and eyespot grana; f, flagella; mg, mastigonemeta of the flagella; r, reservoir; fb, fibrillar system of reservoir; ax, axonemata.

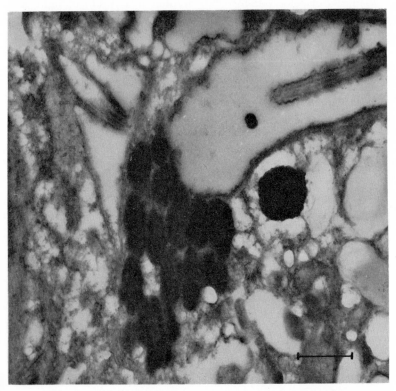

Fig. 31. Electron micrograph of the eyespot of *E. granulata*.

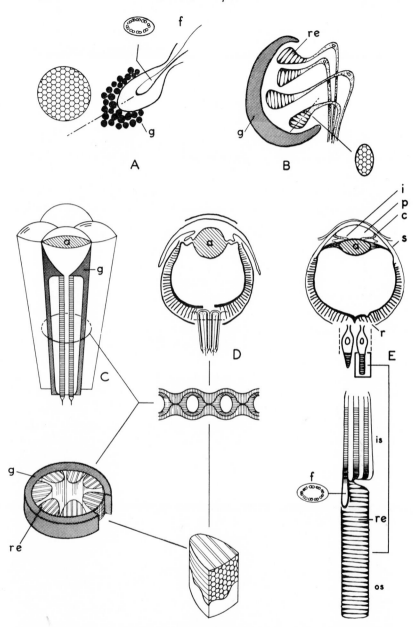

Fig. 32. Schematic development and structure of photoreceptors. A, eyespot of *Euglena*; B, sensory cell of *Planaria*; C, compound eye of insects; D, mollusc cephalopod (*Octopus, Sepia*); and E, vertebrate eye. f, flagellum; g, pigment-screening granules; re, retinal rod structure; os, outer segment; and is, inner segment of the vertebrate retinal rod.

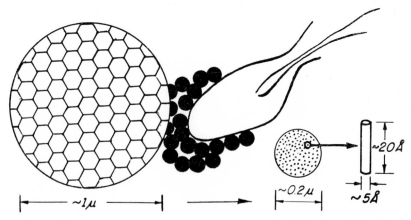

Fig. 33. Schematized packing of eyespot granules (enlargement of Fig. 32A).

found, as in *E. granulata* (Fig. 31). Because of these observations, the *Euglena* eyespot has been likened to the visual photoreceptors. Such a comparison has been drawn schematically in Fig. 32, in which the *Euglena* eyespot can be compared to the invertebrate visual photoreceptors (B-D) and also to the vertebrate retinal rod (E), in which the pigment granules would be analogous to the outer segment and the flagellum to the inner segment of a retinal rod (164a, 165b).

Since we have been unable to clearly resolve the eyespot's fine structure, or identify its photosensitive pigment, any structural molecular model similar to that proposed for the chloroplast would be very speculative. However, based on the fact that the eyespot contains carotenoid molecules, *e.g.*, β-carotene, and on the assumption that they would be packed as monolayers on the surface of these granules, a schematic representation is illustrated in Fig. 33. If the linear carotenoid molecules (5 to 10 Å in diameter) are assumed to be tightly packed and touching on six sides, a rough calculation would then indicate that there would be 5×10^5 to 1×10^6 pigment molecules in the eyespot. There are of the order of 3×10^8 carotenoid molecules in the chloroplasts and 1×10^6 to 1×10^9 retinene (vitamin A aldehyde) molecules found in the retinal rods of the eye. Therefore, the number of the pigment molecules would be of the same order as that found for other photoreceptors.

5 | ENVIRONMENTAL EFFECTS

"Each cell, each living being has a multipotential biochemical personality but the physiochemical environment determines the one under which it manifests itself." (Rene J. Dubos, *Louis Pasteur,* p. 383, Little, Brown and Co., Boston, 1950.)

Euglena grows with or without light, but light is essential for chlorophyll synthesis and hence the chloroplast structure. Although light is the major factor which controls chlorophyll synthesis, temperatures above 33°C and certain drugs, *e.g.,* streptomycin, will interfere with and prevent chlorophyll synthesis (59). The visible spectrum extends generally from 4000 Å to 8000 Å, merging at its lower and upper limits with ultraviolet and infrared radiation. The natural pigments which absorb strongly within this region of visible light are the agents for many photochemical reactions in nature: photosynthesis, phototropism, and vision.

Light ↔ Darkness

The synthesis of pigments in euglenas can be followed when dark-grown organisms are placed in the light to grow. *Euglena* cultures put through the process of adaptation either to darkness or to light were studied spectroscopically for changes in the pigments (169). For example, organisms that were grown in the dark for 7 to 10 days were resuspended in fresh medium and then subjected to continuous light for various time intervals, and conversely, light-grown organisms were subjected to darkness for various time intervals. At these time intervals, the population density as well as their chlorophyll concentrations were determined (Fig. 34). The profound changes undergone by the chloroplasts during the process of dark- or light-adaptation have an obvious chemical counterpart, namely, chlorophyll seems to be degraded when the euglenas are grown in the darkness, and appears to be synthesized rapidly while they readapt themselves to light. The pigment extracts contain, besides chlorophyll, other pigments, mostly carotenoids, which do not necessarily come from the chloroplasts. In Fig. 34b, the absorption curve marked 0 hours is that of an extract obtained from *Euglena* cultured continuously in light for generations. On this curve the various peaks can be identified as belonging to chlorophylls and carotenoids. The peaks around 630 and 660 $m\mu$, for instance, are due to chlorophyll b and a, respectively, while those between 400 and 500 $m\mu$ are produced jointly by carotenoids and chlorophylls. The curve marked 0 hours in Fig. 34a corresponds to the dark-adapted euglenas and indicates that although the organisms look colorless, they still contain a small amount of pigment (pheophytin and the carotenoids). The curves marked 3, 6, and 11 hours show that, when dark-grown organisms are exposed to light, the amount of pigment decreases during the first few hours, which could have some relation to the bleaching of chlorophyll induced by light *in vivo*. After 11 hours, the synthesis overcomes the bleaching, and between 24 and 48 hours a rapid increase in chlorophyll occurs. Fig. 34b illustrates the fate of the pigments in the reverse experiment. The disappearance of chlorophyll seems to be more gradual than its formation, and measurable amounts of chlorophyll and pheophytin persist after days of growth in darkness. Even after chloroplast destruction, some pigment still remains. It is possible that, in darkness, chloroplast remnants containing chlorophyll remain.

The absorption spectra for the light-grown organisms, extracted in acetone, show that the major absorption peaks occur at 663, 615, and 430 $m\mu$, with minor peaks at 580, 536, and 480 $m\mu$. The absorption spectra for dark-adapting organisms show a gradual drop in the intensity of peaks, along with a shift of the maxima from 430 to 410 $m\mu$, from 615 to 605 $m\mu$, and from 536 to 533 $m\mu$, with an increase in intensity, and minor peaks at 555 and 500 $m\mu$, while the 580 $m\mu$ peak becomes a minimum. The time required for this change usually depends upon whether the culture placed in darkness is newly inoculated or whether it has been growing in light for some time.

The effect of darkness on growth and chlorophyll synthesis appears inhibitory to those euglenas grown in light. The individual organisms tend to become small, spherical, and yellowish in color as the time of

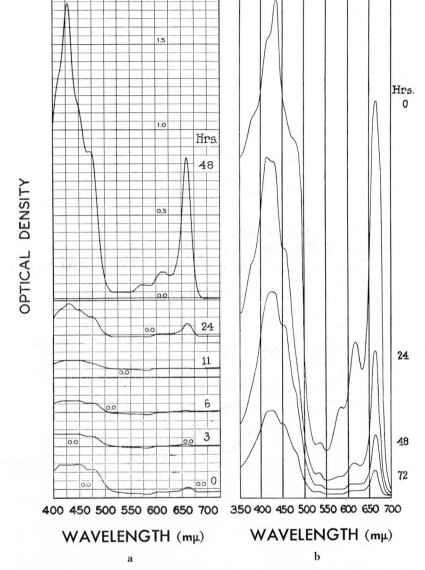

OPTICAL DENSITY

WAVELENGTH (mμ)

a

WAVELENGTH (mμ)

b

Fig. 34. A series of absorption curves (80% acetone-extract of cells). a. Obtained during the adaptation of a culture of colorless *Euglena* to light. b. Illustration of the reverse experiment in which a culture of green *Euglena* was adapted to darkness.

growth in darkness increases. The chlorophyll concentration also decreases as noted in Fig. 34b. This phenomenon has been referred to as "decay"; however, it is not yet known with certainty whether the chlorophyll is actually destroyed or just "diluted." Under the microscope, green granular material could be seen inside the individual organisms which were originally taken from cultures that appeared white, and from which extremely little or no chlorophyll could be extracted. There is a possibility that as the *Euglena* becomes transformed into the spore-like form, some compound impervious to the extracting solvents is formed and prevents the chlorophyll from being extracted.

Extractions from the dark-grown euglenas showed that the concentration began to decrease within 48 hours. However, no change was observed in the spectrum, except for a slight drop in the 580 mμ peak and a slight rise in the 410 mμ peak. Between 48 and 144 hours, a general shift occurred in the absorption spectrum. The absorption maxima at 144 hours agree almost exactly with maxima given by Fischer and Stern (29) for pheophytin, a compound like chlorophyll but lacking magnesium. These changes are typical of the shift from chlorophyll *a* to pheophytin *a*; pheophytin may be formed *in vivo* on many occasions.

It has been known that pheophytin is formed by acid treatment of the chlorophylls. On the possibility that our findings might have been due to conversion of chlorophyll during extraction, we tried washing the concentrated organisms and/or extracting them in acetone buffered with carbonates; no differences were found. Pheophytin may be formed within 24 hours when a culture is placed in the dark. A culture 13 days old in light did *not* form pheophytin appreciably after three months in the dark; a second transfer, six days old in light, handled in the same way at the same time, *did* form pheophytin within 24 hours with no stimulation other than the same transfer to darkness.

Pheophytin appears to be formed when the culture is grown above 40°C; it is possible that some death at this temperature and above may account for the pheophytin found. Pheophytin formation is not, we believe, associated with conversion from motile to palmellar forms. In a light-grown culture adapted up to five hours in the dark, the count of palmellar forms increased greatly while the active forms decreased. After 5 to 24 hours in the dark, the same culture showed a normal growth in count of palmellar forms and almost complete conversion of chlorophyll to pheophytin. Pheophytin formation may be due to a variety of subtle variations concerning the health, disposition, and nutrition of the culture.

Pheophytin is apparently not used in the production of chlorophyll. This agrees with the chemistry of the reactions, where a Grignard reagent is necessary to put magnesium into pheophytin to produce chlorophyll, while simple acid treatment will take it out.

Euglena may lose their ability to synthesize chlorophyll after a long period in the dark. The question arose as to whether the *Euglena* would lose their power to synthesize chlorophyll if they were constantly transferred into fresh medium during their time in the dark. The reversible adaptation of *E. gracilis* from a light photosynthetic organism to a dark chemosynthetic one has been the subject of study by Cramer and Myers (17), Myers (95), and Lwoff (84). We would like to gather here many of our own observations regarding this phenomenon. The change itself is a dramatic one. It can occur within less than 18 hours, or in some cases longer, depending on the previous history of the culture. It is, however, not completely reversible. Some cultures of dark-adapted *Euglena* that had been growing in the dark for longer than 14 days were unable to re-green on adaptation to light; this was evidently a mutation. Other cultures may take a long time in the light before chlorophyll synthesis begins. The pigments which persist in the dark-grown organisms are carotenoids and have been identified as lutein, β-carotene, and neoxanthin (43). (Refer to the discussion of pigments in Chapter 3.)

Light and the Effectiveness of the Spectrum for Pigment Synthesis

Research for the "precursor" of chlorophyll in higher plants stimulated us to search for the "precursor" in Protista using similar techniques. The action spectrum for "greening" in etiolated *Avena* seedlings, as determined by Frank (33), agrees with the absorption spectrum for protochlorophyll as given by Noack and Kiessling (99, 100) and Koski and Smith (71). Studies by Smith *et al.* (138-140) indicate that protochlorophyll is the chlorophyll precursor in higher plants. Chlorophyll synthesis in *Euglena* is light-dependent; in the absence of light no chlorophyll will be synthesized. Because of this, graded light energies can be added, and the effect on pigment synthesis followed.

While the chlorophyll and carotenoid densities were being followed during this study, a decrease in carotenoid density was observed at high light intensities. Previously, Strain (145) had suggested that the carotenoids are involved in chlorophyll formation. He based his suggestion on reports that the spectral bands which are most effective in chlorophyll formation are relatively ineffective in carotenoid formation, since a temporary depression of carotenoids but a steady increase of chlorophyll had been noted in the leaves of *Phaseolus multiflorus* on prolonged light exposure by Rudolph (123) and Seybold and Egle (128, 129). Granick (46) also reported a significant decrease in carotenoid density as Mg vinyl pheoporphyrin is transformed to chlorophyll in a mutant of *Chlorella.* A similar decrease in carotenoid density in oat seedlings has been observed at high light intensities, and it has been suggested that the substance responsible for the carotenoid decrease is a porphyrin-type compound concerned with "esterifying" the porphyrin molecule and converting Mg vinyl pheoporphyrin to protochlorophyll, its phytol ester (34).

The possible relationships between the two plastid pigments (chlorophyll and carotenoids) in *Euglena* have been explored. The organisms were cultured in 100-ml cotton-stoppered Petroff flasks containing 50 ml of medium, in a temperature-controlled room ($25°C \pm 2°C$). The use of the small flat flasks resulted in an even light distribution throughout each culture. The flasks were placed in filter boxes and

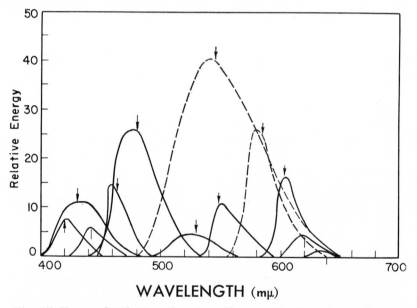

Fig. 35. Energy distribution of various filter combinations. Arrow denotes dominant wavelength. Dotted curves reduced to one-half their height. Curves recorded with the Beckman DK recording spectrophotometer.

exposed to light of different intensities and wavelengths (167, 168). The filters used to vary wavelengths were Klett, Wratten gelatin, and Corning Glass color filters. Energy distribution curves for the various combinations were obtained using a Beckman DK recording spectrophotometer. The light source was a 20 w General Electric fluorescent tube. The intensity of the light varied from 50 to 100 foot-candles depending on the distance of the cultures from the lamp. By substituting the fluorescent tube for the tungsten lamp on the spectrophotometer, energy distribution recordings could be obtained for the filters in terms of the fluorescent lamp output (Fig. 35). The center of gravity of each curve was determined; the wavelength corresponding to the center of gravity was taken as the dominant wavelength of the filter combination. The relative energy of the filter is listed in Table 12. All pigment extractions were carried out in green light.

TABLE 12

RECIPROCAL OF RELATIVE ENERGY FOR A CONSTANT AMOUNT OF CHLOROPHYLL
FORMED AFTER 96 HOURS EXPOSURE TO LIGHT OF DIFFERENT WAVELENGTHS

Filter combinations	Dominant wavelength, $m\mu$	Relative energy	Log relative energy	Chlorophyll formation, per cent	Log relative energy →50 per cent chlorophyll	Relative energy →50 per cent chlorophyll	$\frac{1}{E}$
Corning 3389 + Klett purple	420	11.20	1.0492	31.7	1.345	22.13	0.045
Corning 3060 + Wratten purple	430	14.55	1.1639	51.2	1.140	13.00	0.077
Corning 3389 + 5113	442	8.0	0.9031	20.0	1.470	29.52	0.037
Klett blue	465	18.0	1.2553	23.9	1.735	54.33	0.018
Corning 3387 + 5562	480	36.0	1.5563	53.0	1.525	33.50	0.030
Klett + Wratten green	530	5.5	0.7404	13.8	1.465	29.27	0 034
Corning 3384 + 4303	545	15.2	1.1820	36.9	1.385	34.22	0.041
Corning 3384 + 3385	548	88.8	1.9478	100.0	1.360	23.6	0.042
Corning 3484 + 3480	585	65.0	1.8192	96.1	1.265	18.41	0.054
Corning 2424 + 2434	603	22.9	1.3598	46.1	1.420	26.31	0.038
Corning 2424 + 2412	620	6.2	0.7925	40.4	0.870	7.414	0.135
Corning 2412 + 2404	640	1.4	0.1461	8.5	1.025	10.59	0.094

In evaluating the relative effectiveness of various regions of the spectrum for chlorophyll formation, the method of treating the data was essentially that of Frank (33). It has been shown that chlorophyll synthesis versus energy at two different wavelengths yields parallel curves, as shown in Fig. 36 for the two wavelengths 465 and 586 $m\mu$ (167, 168). The culture which produced the largest amount of chloro-

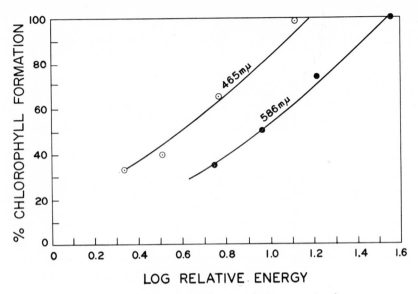

Fig. 36. Chlorophyll formation at different relative energies for two wave-lengths, 96-hour cultures.

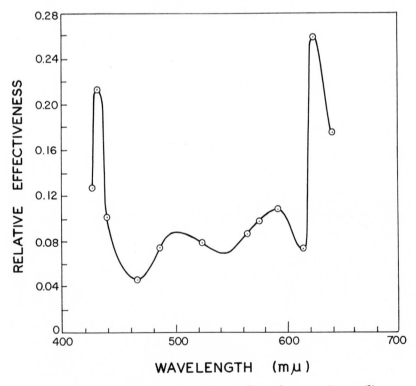

Fig. 37. Action spectrum for chlorophyll synthesis in *E. gracilis*.

phyll was arbitrarily selected as 100 per cent chlorophyll formation. Table 12 lists the reciprocals of the relative energy needed for 50 per cent chlorophyll formation at various wavelengths. From this data, an action spectrum was plotted to which two corrections were made: First, not all light transmitted by any filter is effective in chlorophyll formation, and by multiplying the energy of the filter and the relative energy from the action spectrum at appropriate wavelengths, new energy distribution curves and new dominant wavelengths were obtained for each filter combination. Second, a correction for the number of incident quanta was made by multiplying the reciprocal of the energy from the action spectrum by the energy of the quantum at that wavelength. The resultant curve is an action spectrum given in Fig. 37. It will be noted that the absorption in the blue is lower than in the red, indicating that some pigments, probably the carotenoids which absorb strongly in the blue range, are screening the chlorophyll molecules. This has been demonstrated in albino and normal corn leaves by Koski and Smith (71). In albino leaves, in which only traces of carotenoids are present, a high blue absorption band is found, but in normal leaves, in which carotenoids are in abundance, the absorption in the blue by chlorophyll is lower than in the red.

Chlorophyll concentration increases with the light intensity for a 96 hour exposure. However, carotenoid concentration increases at first and then decreases as the light intensity is increased. The data are given in Table 13 and plotted in Fig. 38. Curves related to the

TABLE 13

CHLOROPHYLL AND CAROTENOID FORMATION IN DARK-ADAPTED
E. gracilis AFTER 96 HOURS' EXPOSURE TO WHITE LIGHT OF
DIFFERENT INTENSITIES

Log relative energy	Chlorophyll density, 663 mμ	Carotenoid density, 475 mμ
1.16	0.023	0.039
1.20	0.024	0.041
1.34	0.028	0.044
1.40	0.029	0.046
1.59	0.035	0.052
1.65	0.037	0.049
1.94	0.047	0.043

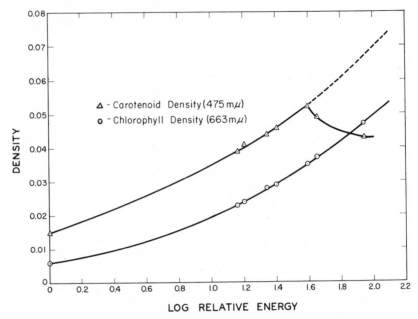

Fig. 38. Effect of increasing intensity of white light on chlorophyll-carotenoid formation in *Euglena*. The dotted extension on the carotenoid curve represents expected carotenoid formation in white light if no destruction had taken place.

action spectra of carotenoid net loss and chlorophyll synthesis can be reconstructed from these data. The greater the amount of pigment formed at a particular wavelength, the greater must be its efficiency. Therefore, by subtracting the density of the pigment formed at one wavelength from the density of the pigment formed in an equal intensity of white light, a value will be obtained the reciprocal of which will be a measure of the effectiveness of that wavelength. This is arrived at by reasoning that the greater the efficiency of the particular wavelength, the smaller will be the difference between the amount of pigment formed at that wavelength and the amount formed in white light. Similar reasoning is applied to the amount of carotenoid formation. The difference between the amount of carotenoid expected to be formed (dotted curve in Fig. 38) in white light and the amount actually formed at a particular wavelength is a direct measure of the effectiveness of that wavelength in carotenoid net removal. The data are recorded in Table 14 and plotted in Figs. 39 and 40.

One must decide what the curve showing effectiveness in carotenoid net removal (Fig. 39) represents. If the same substance is responsible

TABLE 14

Effectiveness of Various Wavelengths in Chlorophyll Formation and in Carotenoid Net Loss over the Expected Gain in White Light

Log relative energy	Dominant wave-length, mμ	"C"$_w$	C$_\lambda$	Δ("C"$_w$ − C$_\lambda$)	$\dfrac{1}{\Delta(\text{"C"}_w - C_\lambda)}$	Cl$_w$	Cl$_\lambda$	Δ(Cl$_w$ − Cl$_\lambda$)	$\dfrac{1}{\Delta(\text{Cl}_w - \text{Cl}_\lambda)}$
1.0492	420	0.036	0.020	0.016	62.5	0.021	0.013	0.008	125.0
1.1639	430	0.039	0.027	0.012	83.3	0.0235	0.018	0.0055	181.8
0.9031	442	0.0325	0.012	0.0205	48.7	0.018	0.008	0.010	100.0
1.2553	465	0.0415	0.014	0.0275	36.3	0.025	0.009	0.016	62.5
1.5563	480	0.051	0.019	0.032	31.2	0.0335	0.017	0.0155	64.6
0.7404	530	0.029	0.010	0.019	52.6	0.015	0.005	0.010	100.0
1.1820	545	0.038	0.020	0.018	55.5	0.023	0.012	0.011	86.9
1.9478	548	0.068	0.041	0.027	37.0	0.0475	0.035	0.0125	80.0
1.8129	585	0.061	0.038	0.026	38.4	0.042	0.034	0.008	125.0
1.3598	603	0.0445	0.023	0.0215	46.5	0.028	0.020	0.008	125.0
0.7925	620	0.030	0.023	0.007	142.8	0.016	0.012	0.004	250.0
0.1461	640	0.017	0.009	0.008	125.0	0.007	0.002	0.005	200.0

C$_\lambda$ = carotenoid density at wavelength λ,

"C"$_w$ = carotenoid density expected at equal intensity of white light,

Cl$_\lambda$ = chlorophyll density at wavelength λ,

Cl$_w$ = chlorophyll density at equal intensity of white light,

$\dfrac{1}{\Delta(\text{Cl}_w - \text{Cl}_\lambda)}$ = effectiveness in chlorophyll synthesis,

$\dfrac{1}{\Delta(\text{"C"}_w - C_\lambda)}$ = effectiveness in carotenoid synthesis,

L$_\lambda$ = effectiveness in carotenoid loss,

$\Delta(\text{"C"}_w - C_\lambda)$ = measure of net effectiveness of the two processes $L_\lambda + \dfrac{1}{\Delta(\text{"C"}_w - C_\lambda)}$.

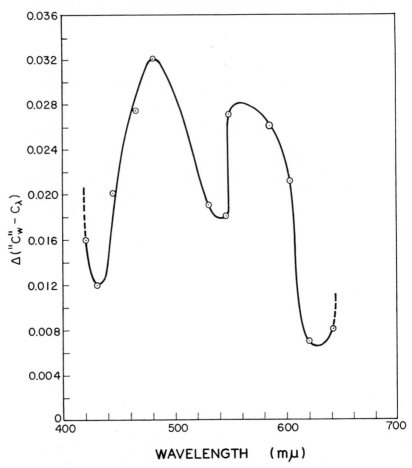

Fig. 39. Reconstructed curve related to the action spectrum of the substance
responsible for carotenoid net removal.

for carotenoid loss and gain, and both are represented in the curve
equally, then their spectral properties should cancel each other. If,
however, the two substances are widely different and enter into the
curve equally, the resultant curve would be meaningless. Neither of
these seems to be the case. If the curve represents mainly the substance concerned with carotenoid removal, the curve itself should
suggest the compound responsible, but the curve does not suggest
any known compound. However, if the curve represents primarily the
substances responsible for carotenoid synthesis, then the reciprocal of
the curve should give the spectral characteristics of that compound.

The reciprocal curve of Fig. 39 is plotted in Fig. 40 along with the curve for chlorophyll formation. It will be observed that the "fit" of the two curves is very close; for this reason, the last assumption appears most plausible.

Is the similarity between the carotenoid synthesis and chlorophyll synthesis curves meaningful? First, the action spectrum for the chlorophyll "precursor" (Fig. 37) should be considered. We have suggested, from the similarity between our action spectrum and the absorption spectrum of protochlorophyll (167, 168), that the precursor in *Euglena* would be protochlorophyll. A substance fluorescing in the range between 520 and 580 mμ was found in the *in vivo* dark-adapted organisms, but no fluorescence was observed in the spectral range of protochlorophyll (635 and 650 mμ). However, based on the absorption maximum (in ether) at 451.5 mμ and a very low peak at 623 mμ,

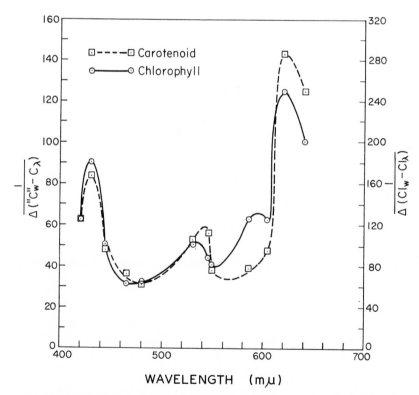

Fig. 40. Reconstructed curves related to the action spectra of the substances responsible for chlorophyll and carotenoid synthesis. The left scale is used with the carotenoid curve and the right scale with the chlorophyll curve.

Nishimura and Huzisige (98) have recently claimed the isolation of protochlorophyll from colorless *E. gracilis* by extraction and chromatography (see Table 15).

TABLE 15

PROTOCHLOROPHYLL FROM VARIOUS SOURCES

Major peaks, mμ	Minor peaks, mμ	Source
650, 445	593, 548	Koski and Smith (71), albino corn seedlings
695, 445	575, 545	Frank (33), oat seedlings
622, 431	590, 510	Wolken and Mellon (167), *Euglena gracilis*
		Absorption spectra for *protochlorophyll* in:
629, 434	578	(a) methanol
623, 432	571, 535	(b) ether

There is every indication that the precursor is a porphyrin-type compound; the wavelength of the absorption bands and the peak ratios of the action spectrum indicate this quite strongly. In addition, mixed etioporphyrins have been extracted from dark-adapted organisms (Fig. 41), using a Granick method (45), but it has not been possible as yet to identify any individual porphyrins. It may be that the conversion of the "precursor" to chlorophyll is so rapid in *Euglena* that the precursor is not built up in sufficient quantity to permit its identification in the normal organisms.

In the absence of isolation, the action spectrum must serve as the most reliable indication of the "precursor," and the action spectrum resembles the absorption spectrum of protochlorophyll more than any other known compound of this type. In Fig. 42, the action spectrum for chlorophyll synthesis is plotted against the relative absorption curve of protochlorophyll in ether solution. The action spectra for protochlorophyll in various plants was also compared with the absorption spectra of protochlorophyll in methyl alcohol and ether as solvents (Table 15). It appears from the absorption peaks that this precursor is protochlorophyll, and from our studies on spectral changes

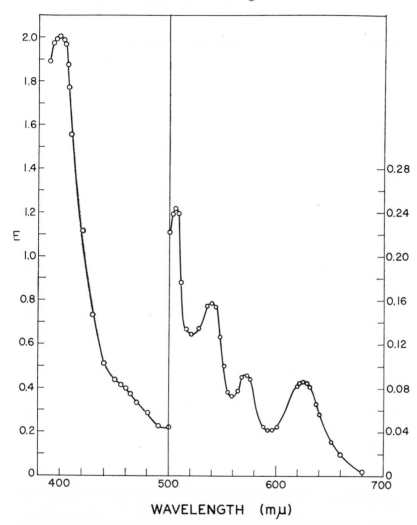

Fig. 41. Absorption spectrum of mixed porphyrins extracted from both dark-adapted *Euglena* and the chlorophyll-free mutant. E signifies relative extinction. The scale on the left is five times that on the right.

from dark-adaptation to light-adaptation, we have been impressed by a decrease of pigment during the first hours of light-adaptation before a rapid synthesis of chlorophyll takes place. On the other hand, this suggests that protochlorophyll may not be the light-acceptor and that another compound, such as Mg vinyl pheoporphyrin a_5, is one of the dark-accumulated precursors. This may also imply that several

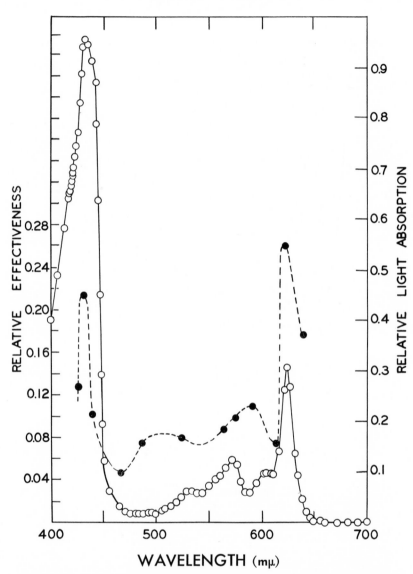

Fig. 42. Comparison of the absorption spectrum of protochlorophyll to the action spectrum of chlorophyll synthesis in *E. gracilis* (———— absorption spectrum of protochlorophyll; ----- action spectrum of protochlorophyll). (Refer to Wolken and Mellon, 167.)

or a group of compounds in the biosynthetic sequence would transfer their energy from one pigment molecule to another pigment molecule.

Frank has reported that carotenoids decrease at high intensities of *both* red and blue light, indicating that the light synthesis of carotenoids is probably not autocatalytic but is influenced by a pigment which absorbs light in both the red and the blue portions of the spectrum (34). Our "action" spectrum for carotenoid synthesis (Fig. 40) seems to substantiate this finding. We have observed the phenomenon of the carotenoid light "destruction" in a chlorophyll-less mutant of *Euglena* which we have recently isolated from our cultures. The mutant, when grown in white light ($\sim$300 foot-candles), produces large quantities of carotenoids for the first two weeks. The color of the culture then fades over the period of a week from a brilliant orange to a yellowish brown. Using a method of Granick, a pale pink pigment was extracted. The absorption spectrum was the same as that obtained with the normal dark-adapted organisms (Fig. 41), again indicating the presence of porphyrins. In addition to the peaks shown, a peak was found at 320 to 330 mμ and another at 230 mμ in the ultraviolet. However, the pigments were present in very low concentration, and no extensive isolation and identification studies could be made.

The curve representing the action spectrum for carotenoid net removal (Fig. 39) is extrapolated in both the blue and red regions of the spectra. The shape of the curve seems to indicate that there might be two other absorption bands, one somewhere in the red and one in the near ultraviolet. Frank has suggested that there may be a porphyrin-like system involved in removing carotenoids and subsequently phytolizing the precursor before its conversion to chlorophyll (34). We have found no evidence of the "phytolization." However, the great decrease in carotenoid concentration in the chlorophyll-free mutant, accompained by a rise in porphyrin concentration, would seem to indicate that the two processes of chlorophyll and carotenoid synthesis are closely related.

Temperature

The general effects of elevated temperatures on the growth of *Euglena* and the bleaching of chlorophyll were investigated. It has been shown that temperature affects chlorophyll synthesis, and that the organism is irreversibly bleached after continuous incubation at temperatures of 32 to 35°C (167, 168). To examine this phenomenon, cultures were grown at 33, 38, 43, 45, and 48°C. In the first 24 hours,

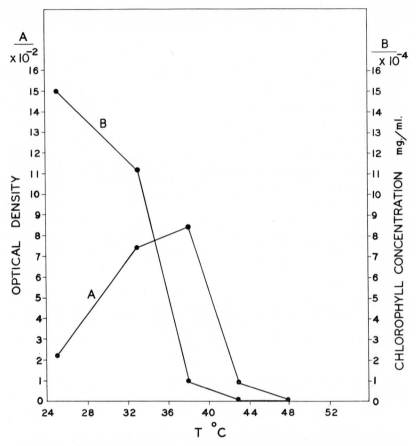

Fig. 43. A. Relative growth after 24 hours exposure at various temperatures.
B. Relative chlorophyll concentration for various temperatures at 24 hours.
Light-grown organisms.

growth increased with temperature up to 38°C. Growth ceased within
the first hour at 43°C. The relative amount of growth after 24 hours'
incubation at various temperatures is shown in Fig. 43, curve A.
Curve B shows the relative amount of chlorophyll in these cultures
after 24 hours. Organisms exposed to temperatures of 43 and 48°C
grew when re-inoculated into fresh media at room temperature, but
were no longer capable of synthesizing chlorophyll in the light. Chlorophyll synthesis increased with temperature to 38°C, at which temperature no new chlorophyll was formed; at 43°C it decreased rapidly
within the first hour, and at 48°C within the first 30 minutes (Fig. 44).

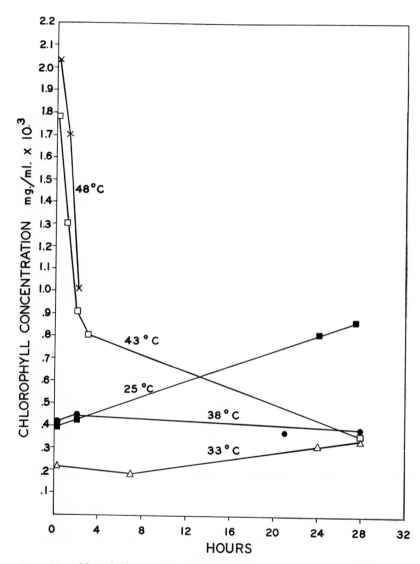

Fig. 44. Chlorophyll concentration at various temperatures (light-grown Euglena).

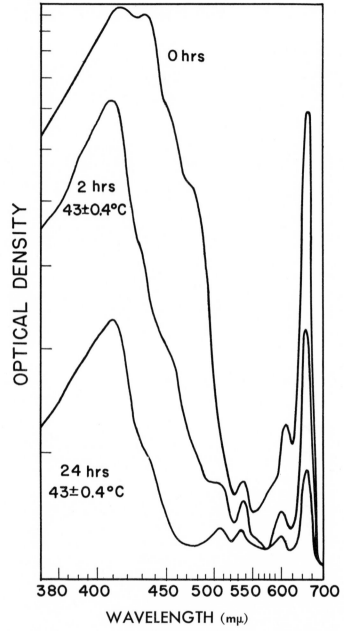

Fig. 45. Absorption spectra for acetone-extract of a 43°C light-grown culture.

These temperature effects were accompanied by structural changes within the chloroplast. After 10 minutes at 45°C, the cytoplasm became very granular with many dense (osmium-fixed) lipid granules. The chloroplasts appeared to be spheres without much structure, and after 20 minutes at 45°C, the chloroplasts had completely broken or collapsed. The absorption spectra of pigment extracts in acetone from 43 and 48°C cultures showed a shift in the major absorption peaks to pheophytin, as was observed in the dark-adapting cultures. This is illustrated in Fig. 45, which shows the absorption spectra for the acetone-extracts of 43°C cultures at various times.

In the light, the rate of chlorophyll synthesis for *Euglena* increases with temperature, as indicated, but degradation of chlorophyll becomes noticeable at 38 and 43°C within an hour, and at 48°C within 30 minutes. In darkness, chlorophyll is bleached at a rate which is independent of the experimental temperatures below 32°C, but at a rate which is temperature-dependent above 32°C. Although it is difficult to study quantitatively the degradation of chlorophyll *in vivo*, data were obtained for the rate of "bleaching" in the first few hours at 33 to 48°C in white light.

In these studies on the irreversible *in vivo* temperature-bleaching of *Euglena* at 33, 38, 40, 43, and 48°C, it was noted that the pH of the cultures varied from 7 to 8 on harvesting the cells, and that the bleached cells showed a replacement of the major chlorophyll absorption peaks to those of pheophytin. These measurements of chlorophyll concentration, calculated from the absorption spectra, are used in Fig. 46 to construct a plot of the log of the concentration (in mg/ml) at various temperatures as a function of time. At a temperature (38°C) closer to the optimum for cellular growth, the concentration of chlorophyll remains almost constant within experimental time. At higher temperatures, bleaching occurs, coupled with general deterioration and ultimate death of the cells. In Fig. 47, the slopes of the lines k_1, k_2, k_3, and k_4 represent reaction rate constants in reciprocal hours. If they are plotted against the reciprocal of absolute temperature, a straight line is obtained. From a straight line drawn through these points in Fig. 47, the activation energy of "bleaching" was calculated, using the three available combinations of k values (k_1, k_2, and k_3); a mean value of 67 k cal/mole was obtained for *Euglena*. If a straight line were drawn through the points k_2, k_3, and k_4, a much higher activation energy would have been calculated.

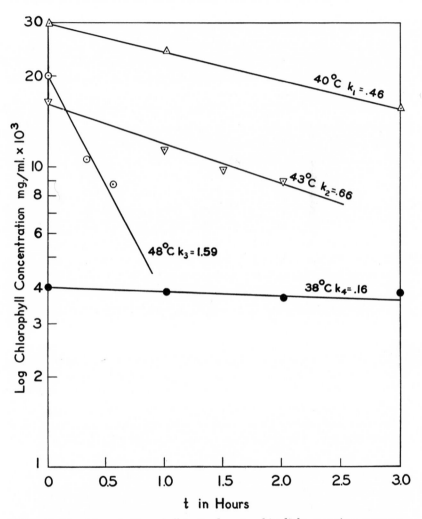

Fig. 46. Bleaching of chlorophyll in *Euglena* in white light at various temperatures. The slopes of these lines, k_1, k_2, k_3, and k_4, are the reaction rate constants in reciprocal hours for each temperature.

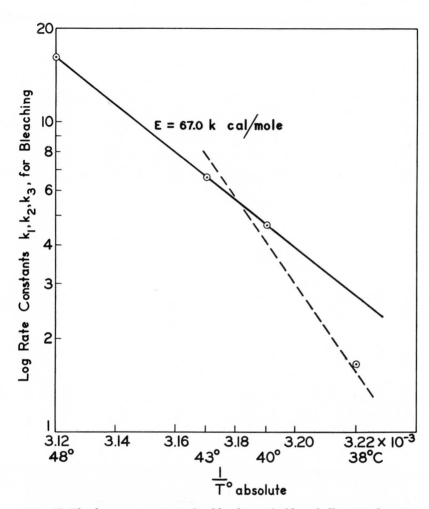

Fig. 47. The log rate constants for bleaching of chlorophyll in *Euglena* in white light plotted against the inverse of the absolute temperature. From the slope of this line, an activation energy of 67.0 k cal/mole has been calculated.

Chloroplastin Bleaching in White Light and Darkness

It is much easier to study the kinetics of the pigment-bleaching in solution than in the living organisms. Thus, for these experiments chloroplastin, the pigment-complex in digitonin, pH 7.2, was used to see whether it would be helpful in learning about the "bleaching" of chlorophyll *in vivo* and the relationship between light- and heat-bleaching. The dry weight of the pigment-complex averaged 28.63 mg/ml, of which 6.06×10^{-5} moles/liter was chlorophyll and 0.36 mg/ml nitrogen.

Petroff flasks (100-ml) were used as the experimental reaction vessels. The entire surface of each flask was painted black, except for

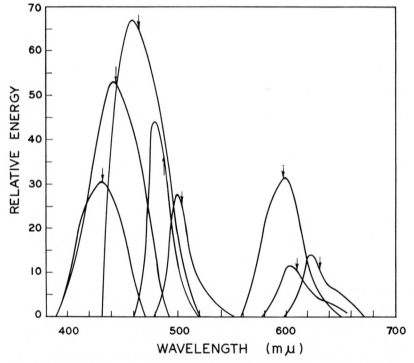

Fig. 48. Effective energy distribution of various filter combinations, obtained by multiplying together (a) the relative energy of the filters, (b) the energy distribution of the light source, and (c) the absorption spectrum of chloroplastin (relative to absorbed energy). The arrows denote the dominant wavelength of each filter combination. The filters are listed in Table 16.

a 16 cm² window on the front, over which various light filter combinations were placed. The relative energy of the filters, the energy distribution of the lamp, and the absorption spectrum of chloroplastin were multiplied together at appropriate wavelengths, and the resulting energy values were plotted against wavelengths for each filter combination in Fig. 48 and in Table 16. To prevent photo-oxidation,

TABLE 16

FILTER COMBINATIONS USED TO STUDY CHLOROPLASTIN BLEACHING

Filter combinations	Center of gravity of the transmission band, mμ	Relative energy transmitted at center of gravity of transmission band, %
Corning 5850 + 5543 *	432	8.0
Corning 9780 (½ thickness) + 5543 *	444	9.0
Corning 3389 + 5562 *	465	10.0
Corning 3385 + 5030 *	487	8.0
Corning 3384 + 9780 *	504	9.0
Corning 3384 + 3480 *	596	8.0
Corning 2424 + 2434	610	8.5
Corning 2412	630	8.5

* Neutral filters were used to reduce the light intensity.

the flasks were flushed with nitrogen before and after the addition of 50 ml of chloroplastin. Bleaching was measured in terms of decrease in optical density or increase in percentage transmission of the chloroplastin with time, at 675 mμ. The absorption spectra of the bleached chloroplastin preparations are illustrated in Fig. 49.

In white light, at 10, 30, and 40°C, the bleaching rate of chloroplastin is practically independent of temperature (Fig. 50). In darkness at 30°C, the increase in transmission of the chloroplastin preparation is less than 6 per cent in 24 hours, but bleaching is rapid when the temperature is raised to 40°C. The ratio between the rates of

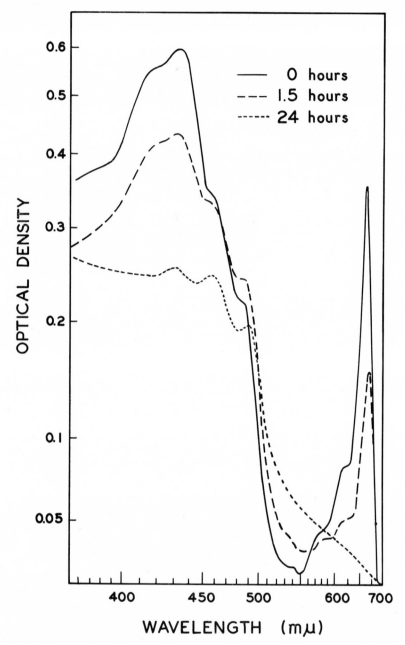

Fig. 49. Bleaching of chloroplastin in white light at 25°C. Extract prepared from light-grown *Euglena* in 1.8 per cent digitonin, pH 7.2.

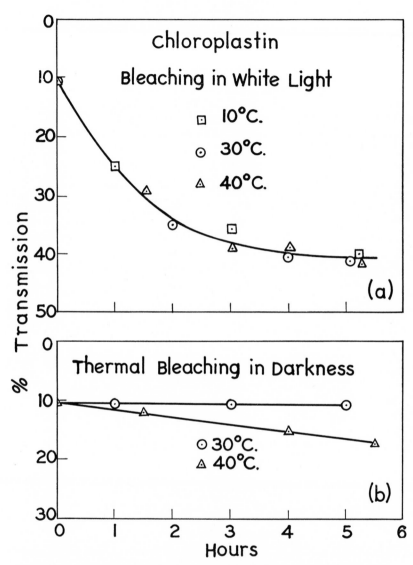

Fig. 50. (a) Chloroplastin bleaching in white light at various temperatures. (b) Thermal bleaching of chloroplastin in darkness. Bleaching measured as increase in percentage of transmission, at 675 mμ, of the chloroplastin (pH 7.2) with time.

bleaching at 30 and 40°C, or Q_{10}, is 13.25. The activation energy of the thermal bleaching of chloroplastin is calculated by applying Arrhenius' equation:

$$\frac{d \ln k}{dT} = \frac{E}{RT^2}$$

where k is the rate constant, T the absolute temperature, E the activation energy, and R the gas constant. The calculated value was 48.2 k cal/mole. The equation used in the calculation was in the form:

$$\ln \frac{k_2}{k_1} = \frac{E}{R} \frac{T_2 - T_1}{T_1 T_2}$$

Temperature Dependence of Bleaching in Monochromatic Light. The chloroplastin was bleached at various wavelengths at 10 and 30°C. Typical bleaching curves are illustrated in Fig. 51. It can be seen that the k_2/k_1 ratio is ~1 at 504 mμ and slightly <1 at 432 mμ. At 596 and 630 mμ, however, the bleaching rate is higher at the higher tem-

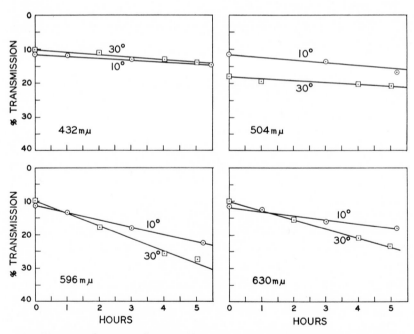

Fig. 51. Typical curves showing bleaching rates of chloroplastin at various wavelengths. No temperature-dependence is found in the bleaching rate below 504 mμ, but high temperature-dependence can be noted at 596 mμ and 630 mμ.

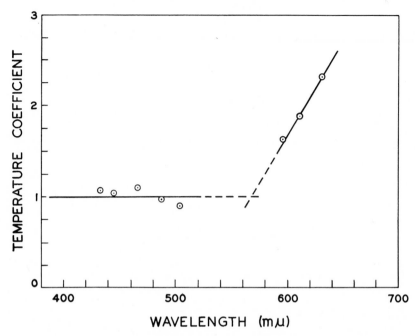

Fig. 52. Temperature-dependence of the bleaching rate of chloroplastin expressed as a function of wavelength. The intersection of the straight lines drawn through the experimental points indicates that temperature-dependence begins at about 560 mμ.

perature. The temperature-dependence of the rate as a function of wavelength is shown in Fig. 52. (Due to the low absorption of chloroplastin at 520 to 580 mμ, no measurements could be made in that region.) Bleaching becomes temperature-dependent at about 560 mμ. The quantum energy at 560 mμ corresponds to about 48.3 k cal, which is equal to the activation energy calculated above for thermal bleaching in darkness. The thermal dependence of bleaching increases with wavelength (Table 17). The total activation energy is the sum of the quantum energy and the thermal activation energy (as calculated from the Arrhenius equation). This sum is found to remain constant from 560 mμ into the red.

The chlorophyll of *Euglena* can be "bleached" by growth in darkness, and in light at temperatures above 33°C. Studies of the chlorophyll bleaching in alcohol or acetone solutions cannot easily be related to the reactions in photosynthesis, since it is necessary to imitate the conditions in the cells more closely. The bleaching as observed

TABLE 17

ACTIVATION ENERGY OF CHLOROPLASTIN BLEACHING

Wave-length, $m\mu$	Q_{20}	Arrhenius energy k cal/mole	Quantum energy k cal/mole	Total energy k cal/mole
Dark	—	48.0	—	48.0
504	0.67	−3.36	52.8	49.4
596	1.46	3.26	44.6	47.9
610	1.54	3.73	43.6	47.3
630	2.01	6.02	42.3	48.3

here was not due to photo-oxidation, since the chloroplastin was in an atmosphere of nitrogen. The bleaching of chloroplastin can be produced by light, heat, or a combination of both. Below 560 $m\mu$, bleaching is accomplished by light energy alone; above 560 $m\mu$, it requires the combined effects of light and heat (167). The total activation energy of bleaching is the same in darkness and in light. The value of 67 k cal/mole calculated for the bleaching *in vivo* is higher than for the chloroplastin-extract. Both, however, are within the range of values that have been found for denaturation of proteins (66).

Since the function of photoreceptors (photosynthetic or visual) is to "trap" light energy for transfer to chemical or electrical energy, and since there is a similarity in structure of the photoreceptors as well as in the pigment-extract in digitonin, it is interesting to compare the light- and heat-bleaching of chloroplastin with that of the visual pigment complex, rhodopsin. Rhodopsin has been shown by Lythgoe and Quilliam (82) to bleach by both light and heat. Rhodopsin bleaches rapidly in the dark at temperatures of 50°C and above, and an activation energy of 44 k cal/mole has been calculated for its bleaching in neutral solutions. St. George (126) showed that the bleaching of rhodopsin in light becomes temperature-dependent at about 590 $m\mu$. He calculated an activation energy of 48.5 k cal/mole for bleaching in the light. When the quantum energy decreases below 48.5 k cal/mole—the energy of the quantum at 590 $m\mu$—the temperature coefficient increases in the same way as we noted for chloroplastin above 560 $m\mu$. We are not implying that these are one and the same mechanism, but only note another comparative similarity for the minimal experimental activation energies for bleaching chloroplastin and rhodopsin (Table 18).

TABLE 18

COMPARISON OF THE BLEACHING OF CHLOROPLASTIN AND RHODOPSIN

	Comparative rate of bleaching at all temperatures in white light	Calculated experimental activation for bleaching in darkness	Experimental wavelength at which temperature dependence begins, mμ	Calculated experimental activation energy for bleaching in light
Chloroplastin, E. gracilis	1	48.2 k cal/mole	560	48.3 k cal/mole
Rhodopsin, frog, cattle	1	44.0 k cal/mole	590	48.5 k cal/mole.

To understand the complete process of bleaching, it is necessary to know more of the mechanism involved; it appears that there would probably be more than one independent mechanism involved in transferring and transforming the light and heat energy.

Metals

The inclusion or omission of various chemical nutrients and metallic ions in the growth medium will also cause noticeable changes in the morphology and the pigments of *Euglena*. Because of this, the effect of metals on growth and pigment synthesis is of considerable importance. Of the metals investigated, magnesium was of greatest interest to us, since as already noted it is necessary for chlorophyll, being the nucleus of the chlorophyll molecule; there is one atom of magnesium per molecule of chlorophyll. Magnesium is also a constituent of the enzyme phosphatase, which plays an important part in phosphate metabolism, and carboxylase, an enzyme that degrades keto-acids. Vitamin B_{12}, a specific requirement of *E. gracilis* for growth, contains one atom of cobalt per molecule and is also a porphyrin-like molecule similar to chlorophyll.

It has been observed in other photosynthetic microorganisms that magnesium deficiency depresses photosynthesis in the light-limited and light-saturated states, as well as in CO_2-limited states. Changes in magnesium concentration affect the chlorophyll concentration of *Chlorella,* in a concentration range in which there is little effect on the rate of photosynthesis. The rate of the dark reaction is also affected by magnesium deficiency, as has been shown from studies of flashing light experiments in photosynthesis.

A magnesium-deficient medium was prepared by omitting all magnesium salts from the standard medium. It was found that growth in the light in the magnesium-deficient environment, as measured by increase in optical density, was not considerably decreased, and in darkness the growth was reduced to one-half of what is normally found. However, the total number of organisms in the complete medium and in the magnesium-deficient medium was the same. Optical density as a measure of growth was misleading in this case, for what resulted was an increase in the total size of the euglenas but not in the number of euglenas.

The formation of large cells and the cessation of cell division was also observed in magnesium-deficient media for the photosynthetic alga *Chlorella* by Finkle and Appleman (28), as well as that for the protozoan *Tetrahymena geleii* grown synthetically by Kidder (70). For *Tetrahymena,* essentially no growth results when magnesium is omitted from the medium; with the addition of magnesium (as the salt $MgSO_4 \cdot 7H_2O$), growth is restored to half-maximal. After three transfers in magnesium-deficient medium, *E. gracilis* became spherical, averaging $8 \times 10 \; \mu$ in size, and became almost colorless. The rate of growth was slow and was one-fourth of that in a standard complete medium. Absorption spectra of Mg^{++}-deficient and metal-deficient cells extracted in acetone are shown in Fig. 53. The addition of small traces of magnesium to the *E. gracilis* culture had a considerable effect on growth and pigment synthesis, and all the organisms were moderately active.

Radioactive magnesium, Mg^{28}, with a half-life of 22 hours, which is considered a long half-life for magnesium, was used to determine the degree to which magnesium is incorporated or exchanged in the growing cells and in the synthesis of chlorophyll molecules. The radioactive magnesium was placed into our growth media as an inorganic salt, and its uptake in the organisms and various cell fractions was determined as a function of time, growth of new cells, and chlorophyll molecules synthesized. We anticipated information relative to the num-

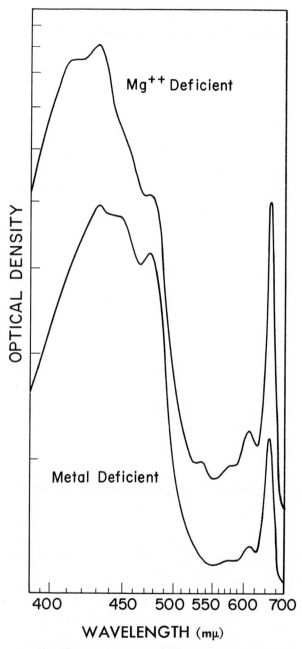

Fig. 53. Absorption spectra of 85 per cent aqueous acetone-extracts of Mg-deficient cultures grown in light.

ber of newly formed chlorophyll molecules. Unfortunately, little could be learned about the time in the biochemical events when the magnesium was inserted into the chlorophyll molecules.

The organisms were grown in a metal-free medium from which all the metals (magnesium, molybdenum, cobalt, copper, zinc, iron, manganese, and boron) were omitted. In spite of the fact that all the trace metals cannot be removed by using double-distilled water and ion-exchange resins, they are still referred to as metal-deficient or metal-free media. It was found that complete metal deficiency produces enlargement of the euglena cells and retardation of cellular division (164). This is accompanied by the disintegration of the chloroplast, similar to Mg^{++} deficiency alone, as well as spectral shifts in the chlorophyll, indicative of pheophytin.

Euglenas from a magnesium-deficient culture were inoculated into a metal-free medium and were continually transferred into magnesium-deficient media. The euglenas became small, spherical organisms 10 μ in diameter; they contained granular material but no discernible chloroplasts. A survey of possible metal contaminants from the other ingredients of the medium showed that only an insignificant amount of metal contamination was present in the metal-free medium. In one liter of metal-free medium, there was present a contamination of 50 μg of magnesium. This will perhaps account for the fact that the metal-free cultures green slightly.

Response to Various Metallic Ions. To evaluate the response to various metallic ions, flasks of metal-free medium were prepared and into each of these was placed a single addition of metallic sulfates in the same concentration in which they are present in the standard medium. The metallic ions used were: magnesium, molybdenum, boron, manganese, zinc, copper, and cobalt. A control flask remained metal-free and was used for comparison. Composite graphs of growth and chlorophyll concentration may be seen in Fig. 54. It will be noted from the slopes of the response curves that growth is accelerated more with magnesium than with molybdenum and boron. Manganese, copper, zinc, and cobalt ions were all inhibitory to growth and chlorophyll synthesis, whereas magnesium, molybdenum, and boron stimulated chlorophyll synthesis, in that order.

Microscopic observations showed many morphological differences. In the cultures containing cobalt, copper, manganese, and zinc, the predominating forms were small spore forms, 3×4 μ in size, and dead cells. A very few active *Euglena*, containing eyespots, were seen in the copper and manganese cultures. In the boron, molybdenum,

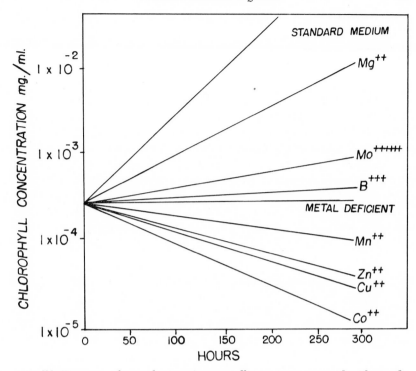

Fig. 54. Response of growth to various metallic ions as compared with standard medium.

and metal-free cultures, the organisms contained green granular material but were reduced in size ($\sim 10 \times 15\ \mu$) compared to an active
Euglena. In the molybdenum medium, a few spore-like forms were
found, but no eyespots could be seen. In cultures with magnesium
present, however, large elongated, active *Euglenas* with discernible
eyespots and chloroplasts predominated.

To find out whether response to metals would be different if the
metals were added as chelates instead of salts, the chelating agent
ethylenediaminetetraacetic acid (EDTA) was used. EDTA may induce deficiencies for several metals. By addition of the metals in question in suitable preparations, this difficulty may be overcome. As the
growing organisms absorb metals (presumably because their surface
is provided with chelating groups which can compete with the exoge-
nous complex formed), more metal ions disassociate from the complex
in compliance with the law of mass action. By this means, dense
growth may be obtained, whereas, if the chelating agent were not

present, the metal concentration needed to secure this growth would be such that precipitation or toxicity might inhibit growth altogether. The metals magnesium, cobalt, manganese, molybdenum, boron, zinc, copper, and iron were added singly to culture flasks of metal-free media containing EDTA. The metals and EDTA were present in the same concentration as in the standard medium. It was found that *Euglena* were able to utilize magnesium, cobalt, manganese, copper, boron, and molybdenum for growth, but not manganese, iron, or zinc as chelates. Chlorophyll synthesis followed essentially the same pattern as growth. Although the euglenas were not able to use Mg^{++} alone as a chelate for growth, there was little or no effect on chlorophyll synthesis. The organisms were able to synthesize chlorophyll equally well whether Mg^{++} was added as a salt or as a chelate. Considerable study is still needed to elucidate the effects of trace metals on growth and pigment synthesis in *Euglena*.

Drug and Radiation Effects

Drug action in cells, like so many other biological phenomena, is difficult to unravel. A drug may inhibit one process yet accelerate another; concentration dependence is always critical, and the reaction can go either way. Firstly, in designing these experiments, only those drugs which were thought to have a specific effect on the biochemistry of pigment synthesis, without inducing cellular death, were searched for. Secondly, it was thought that certain drugs could be found that would have a specificity for the cell membrane, nucleus, eyespot, chloroplast, and other organelles of *Euglena*, that could easily be observed or measured. A good many cellular poisons have a marked effect on photosynthesis. Such poisons as mercuric ion, hydroxylamine, cyanide, and azide are inhibitors of photosynthesis as well as other cellular processes. It has already been indicated that elevated temperatures, metals, and drugs such as streptomycin have a profound effect on pigment synthesis, particularly on chlorophyll and the chloroplast structure.

It is of interest to summarize here some of these experimental drug effects on *Euglena*.

Streptomycin. Some ideas on the mode of action of the antibiotic streptomycin have been discussed by Hutner and Provasoli (60). Streptomycin is believed to interfere with the reaction between pyruvic and oxalacetic acids in the Krebs Cycle, a reaction which seems to be essential for all forms of life. In the animal cells, this reaction is localized in the mitochondria. With the finding that the antibiotic streptomycin preferentially disrupts the synthesis of chlorophyll pigments, and hence the structure of the chloroplast, an attack on the site of photosynthesis became available. Hutner and Provasoli reported that with sensitive *E. gracilis bacillaris* strains as little as 40 μg/ml brought about practically complete chlorophyll destruction in 15 days; 1.0 μg/ml caused an average reduction in "greenness" to half the normal value. Other strains, however, are more resistant to streptomycin bleaching. In our strains of *E. gracilis,* concentrations of 1×10^{-3} to 2.5 mg/ml of streptomycin were employed. At a concentration of 0.2 mg/ml, euglenas with little chlorophyll and a reduced amount of carotenoids were observed, although the growth rate was not much less than expected for normal growth. This bleaching of chlorophyll indicated a shift to pheophytin. At the highest concentration used, 65 per cent of the chlorophyll was "bleached" within 70 hours. Exposure to streptomycin in a concentration of 1 mg/ml decreased the concentration of chlorophyll with time for 15 days (Fig. 55). Streptomycin had the same effect on chlorophyll synthesis as incubation of the culture at 35°C for eight days.

A completely achlorophyllous *Euglena* culture was not obtained at any of these concentrations. It was observed that at all these concentrations of streptomycin the chloroplasts swelled, and many palmelloid forms appeared after 24 hours of growth. All the active forms, though, still contained pigmented eyespots. The electron micrographs of fixed euglenas showed an inflated chloroplast along with the enlargement of the nucleus and endosome. There was still considerable internal structure left in the chloroplast, although some collapsed chloroplasts were observed. These broken and collapsed chloroplasts were similar to those observed in dark-adapted and metal-depleted euglenas. Warburg studies on the streptomycin-treated organisms grown in light revealed that they have a significantly higher level of CO_2 utilization than cells which were shielded from the light, indicating that light does have a definite residual effect which might well be the result of photosynthetic reactions, because the chlorophyll concentration is never completely reduced.

Pyribenzamine. An antihistamine (2-benzyl-2-dimethylaminoethyl-amino-pyridine hydrochloride) is another drug that has a specific effect on pigment synthesis. Gross (50) found pyribenzamine to inhibit chlorophyll synthesis in a similar manner to streptomycin, and colorless mutants were obtained. In a chlorophyll-free mutant isolated from a culture after 33 days' exposure to pyribenzamine, still viable

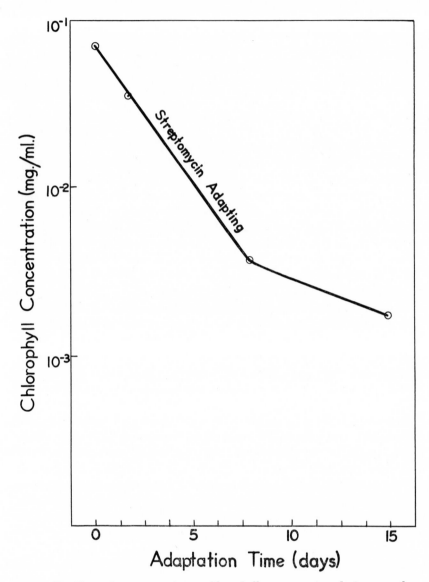

Fig. 55. Effect of streptomycin on chlorophyll concentration during growth.

E. gracilis organisms were observed. In addition, there were some changes in the carotenoid pigments. It should be noted that Goodwin (41) found that diphenylamine interferes with carotenoid synthesis in some organisms, with little reduction in growth.

Colchicine. Colchicine has been found to be generally ineffective on algae and protozoa. *Euglena* appears to be sensitive to some concentrations of about 4 per cent colchicine, and some temporary changes in the chloroplast were noted. However, mitosis and general cellular activity were unaffected by this concentration of colchicine (75). It is believed that the resistance of these organisms stems from the inability of colchicine to penetrate the cell pellicle or membrane.

Barbital. Barbiturates can be considered toxic to humans, especially so in the disease known as *porphyria,* the excretion of porphyrins. It was thought that some noticeable effects would be observed in the pigment synthesis of *Euglena.* In concentrations of 0.01 to 10 mg/ml, no distinguishable changes in the chlorophyll could be detected. At concentrations greater than 0.1 mg/ml, rounding-up and many palmelloid forms were observed.

Azaserine. Recent studies of azaserine and DON (6-diazo-5-oxo-l-norleucine) have been brought to our attention by those who synthesize chemotherapeutic drugs for cancer studies. Azaserine is soluble in water and stable at pH 6.5 for several days. Also it was indicated that azaserine may block some important metabolic pathways in the photosynthetic *Chlorella;* a rather specific antimetabolic effect on the carbon dioxide fixation pattern in algae has been observed (6). In the initial observation, it was implicated as a specific inhibitor of some stages in the metabolic pathways leading to purine and/or pyrimidine synthesis. The effects of azaserine on the path of carbon in photosynthesis by *Scenedesmus* has led to the recognition of a more general, but still inhibitory function. Such studies may give us further information concerning the second and ultimate fate of carbon, initially incorporated via the photosynthetic cycle.

Growth of *Escherichia coli* is inhibited by concentrations of 0.1 to 1.08 μg/ml of azaserine, although less effectively in a complex synthetic medium. It is known that these activities are reversed by various metabolites, including purines and aromatic amino acids. *Euglena* was grown in alkaline media, pH 6.5 to 7.0. From .05 to 5.0 mg/ml of azaserine was added to each culture. It was observed that the growth of *E. gracilis* at these concentrations was inhibited, and at concentrations greater than 5 mg/ml, death resulted. There were also shifts in the chlorophyll absorption peaks to pheophytin. Other drugs are known that will inhibit pigment synthesis; they also cause death of the organisms.

Radiation. Very little interpretable data is available for ultraviolet and x-irradiation of the euglenoids. It is expected that radiation would produce interesting mutants for the study of pigment synthesis. Such studies have been made on other algae and on the euglenoid *Astasia* (126a, 127). So far, too few mutants have been isolated. It has been found that the ultraviolet at 265 mμ is a most effective killing wavelength for *Euglena*. The presence of the chloroplasts does not appear necessary for ultraviolet inactivation. For the same effect to be noted with x-rays as with ultraviolet, it required 20,000 r for 24 hours. The ability of ultraviolet to produce changes in growth and pigment synthesis without killing is presently under study (80). The protozoans investigated for x-ray sensitivity indicate that the flagellates are most radiosensitive, with the possible exception of some colonial forms and the amoebas. A comparative study of protozoan x-ray sensitivity of the flagellates, ciliates, and amoebas has been done by Wichterman and Honegger (161, 162). For a lethal dose, LD$_{50}$ of *E. gracilis* required 32,000 r for 24 hours. Radiation in doses up to 100,000 r had no effect on mitosis and cell activity (75). *Euglena* which were irradiated for 100 minutes for a total of 180,000 r and transferred to a fresh medium showed no apparent immediate effect, but the general growth of the culture was considerably delayed and the organisms were sluggish with many palmelloid forms. They appeared to be resistant to neutron bombardment; 5,000 units were applied to a young culture of *Euglena* with little killing effect, but definite effects were noted after 48 hours' growth (87).

Obviously, too few studies have been made on the toxicity of drugs and on radiation of euglenoids. What is indicated from these few experiments is that there is too little quantitative data available at present to permit any theory on mode of action.

Chemical Analysis

The morphological changes due to environment (light, darkness, temperature, and depletion of metals) are reflected by total gross chemical changes (other than those already noted for the pigments) in *Euglena*. It has been indicated by many researchers that changes in environment produce internal biochemical changes in the organism. From information obtained in chemical analyses, the nature of some of these changes became more evident. As indicated by the analysis in Table 19, the dark-grown *Euglena* and the heat-mutants accumulate carbohydrates and synthesize less protein (about one-half that of the light-grown organisms). These results follow the same pattern as illustrated by the analysis of another photosynthetic alga, *Chlorella.*

TABLE 19

Synthesis of Various Products by Light-Grown and Dark-Grown *Euglena* and *Chlorella*

Product	E. gracilis v. bacillaris				Chlorella	
	Light-grown	Dark-grown	Mg^{++}-deficient (light-grown)	40°C heat-treated (light-grown)	Full light	Weak light
Ash	10.0	8.0	12.1	7.5	10.0	9.0
Fat	13.7	9.1	6.4	7.8	12.0	10.0
Protein	69.3	36.3	73.9	48.1	70.0	46.0
Carbohydrates	7.0	46.6	7.6	36.6	8.0	35.5
Water	77.1	71.4	90.4	77.7	—	—

6

PHOTOSYNTHESIS, RESPIRATION, AND PHOTOCHEMICAL ACTIVITY

"In photosynthesis we are like travelers in an unknown country around whom the early morning fog slowly begins to rise, vaguely revealing the outlines of the landscape. It will be thrilling to see it in bright daylight!" (E. I. Rabinowitch, *The Physics and Chemistry of Life*, Simon and Schuster, New York, 1955.)

Comparative Photosynthesis

A brief discussion of the comparative aspects of photosynthesis, particularly recent studies with photosynthetic bacteria, may be helpful in the clarification of the experiments with *Euglena*. It is not the purpose here to review the whole of photosynthesis since references have already been made to extensive sources. However, it is desirable to indicate, if possible, how the utilization of *Euglena* fits into the general problem (149).

Autotrophic organisms can obtain their energy requirements for growth from sources other than organic molecules; photo-autotrophs derive this necessary energy from light radiation; chemo-autotrophs, from oxidizable inorganic chemicals. The photo-autotrophs fall into three separate groups: green plants, pigmented sulfur bacteria, and pigmented non-sulfur bacteria. These reactions, mediated by light, can be expressed by the following equations:

(a) Green plants—

$$CO_2 + H_2O \xrightarrow{\text{light}} \underset{\text{organic matter}}{(CH_2O)} + O_2 \uparrow$$

(b) Non-sulfur bacteria—

$$CO_2 + \text{Succinate} \xrightarrow{\text{light}} (CH_2O) + \text{fumarate}$$

(c) Sulfur bacteria—

$$CO_2 + H_2S \xrightarrow{\text{light}} (CH_2O) + S$$

For non-sulfur bacteria, the organic donor (succinate) can be substituted for by many different organic acids which have two electrons to spare. For the sulfur bacteria, H_2S can be substituted for by: $Na_2S_2O_3$, $Na_2S_4O_7$, H_2, $S \rightarrow H_2SO_4$, or H_2Se.

This general characterization of the various types of photosynthesis has led to the formulation by van Neil (154) of what is known as the "comparative biochemistry of photosynthesis." In general:

$$CO_2 + H_2A \xrightarrow{\text{light}} (CH_2O) + A$$

Actually, the reaction can be generalized even further. The photosynthetic light reaction can be demonstrated without involving carbon dioxide. In the Hill reaction, quinone or ferric ion can accept the hydrogens which are activated by the light reaction, so the general formula can be written:

$$B + H_2A \xrightarrow{\text{light}} BH_2 + A$$

or simply as a light-induced oxidation-reduction reaction, which requires light energy.

Since the concept has been established that the photochemical reaction in green plant photosynthesis is a photolysis of water, the question arises as to whether some substance, such as H_2S, might perhaps be the activated material in bacterial photosynthesis. The experimental evidence indicates that water is photolyzed in both plant and bacterial photosynthesis. A more acceptable equation for the bacterial systems would include both water and a general hydrogen donor and exclude oxygen evolution. For example:

$$CO_2 + 2H_2A + H_2O \xrightarrow{\text{light}} (CH_2O) + 2H_2O + 2A$$

A simple formulation for the mechanism of the over-all process is yet to be conceived. However, different aspects are reasonably well understood.

The general photosynthetic light reaction can be represented schematically as:

$$HOH \xrightarrow[\text{org.}]{\text{light}} \begin{cases} [H] \xrightarrow[\text{carriers}]{\text{electron transport}} (CH_2O) \\ [OH] \xrightarrow[\text{organic peroxides}]{\text{via } O_2 \text{ carriers}} H_2O + O_2 \text{ or oxidized material} \end{cases}$$

While considering the photosynthetic bacteria, it might be well to discuss the carotenoid function in the primary photosynthetic reaction. All photosynthetic organisms have some type of chlorophyll and two or more carotenoids, all of which are considered to be necessary for photosynthesis. The bacterial systems are unique in being anaerobic and not evolving oxygen. Stanier, at the University of California, has studied the bacterial pigment mutants from the standpoint of photosynthesis and growth (141). Three classes of mutants were obtained from the normal wild type:

Purple—normal wild—bacteriochlorophyll + red and yellow carotenoids

Green—mutant—bacteriochlorophyll + two new yellow carotenoids

Brown—mutant—bacteriochlorophyll + three carotenoids (two wild and one new)

Blue-green—mutant—bacteriochlorophyll + no colored carotenoids (colorless phytoene-saturated C_{40})

The blue-green mutant has been studied extensively because it grows well photosynthetically without the carotenoids which had been considered necessary. However, when the illuminated cultures are exposed to oxygen, very rapid death and bacteriochlorophyll decomposition occur, which are not characteristic of the normal, purple type. This mutant and the normal purple wild type are comparable with respect to concentration of bacteriochlorophyll, carotenoids or their colorless precursors, and photosynthetic rate under anaerobic conditions—demonstrating that the light-trapping process is not dependent on carotenoids if oxygen is not present. Chlorophyll appears to be the only pigment necessary for the primary light reaction.

A direct relationship between the synthetic pathways of both chlorophyll and carotenoids has been shown by action spectra in our studies (167) and by others using different methods. This is not difficult to reconcile with the lack of carotenoids in the blue-green bacterial mutant. The relationship between these two classes of pigments is probably that the C_{20} phytol chain on chlorophyll is derived from precursors of C_{40} and C_{20} carotenoids; and the mutant does have the C_{40} carotenoid precursor, phytoene, which can give rise to the phytol chain via a divergent pathway. The carotenoid synthetic pathway beyond phytoene is genetically blocked in the mutant.

Since its life and integrity are so dependent on the absence of either oxygen or light, the blue-green mutant clearly exhibits the phenomenon of photodynamic action. Photodynamic action refers to the light-sensitization of a biological system by some light-absorbing molecule which becomes activated and causes destructive photo-oxidation. A thorough analysis of the mutant photosynthetic system has disclosed that the bacteriochlorophyll itself is the photosensitized compound and that it is also one of the substances photo-oxidized. Therefore, the carotenoids somehow protect the light-sensitized chlorophyll from self-destructive oxidation. Similarly, Sager and Zalokar have indicated, from their studies of a pale green mutant of the alga *Chlamydomonas reinhardi* (125), that the carotenoids are not essential, except in catalytic amounts, for green plant photosynthesis, but are probably necessary for protection against photodynamic destruction.

The bacterial chromatophores contain the pigments, bacteriochlorophyll, and carotenoid molecules, complexed with lipoprotein (or protein) in some order of molecular organization. Since the blue-green mutant lacks the rigid carotenoid molecules, but contains the less rigid phytoene, the mutant chromatophores probably have a more "loosely" organized structure. If we associate a highly organized internal structure with photosynthetic efficiency, the mutant is only about 75 per cent as efficient as the wild type.

The universal occurrence of carotenoids in all autotrophic plants indicates that it must play some part in photosynthesis. Fujimori and Livingston (36) recently studied the interactions of chlorophyll *in vitro* in its triplet state, with oxygen and carotene, and found that β-carotene quenches the triplet state as strongly as does oxygen and that it has no noticeable effect upon the amount of fluorescence of chlorophyll *b*. It has been demonstrated that the Hill reaction is inhibited if the carotene (but not the chlorophyll) is extracted from a chloroplast preparation. These investigations give some support to the view that carotene plays a direct part in the primary act of photosynthesis. It is reasonable to speculate that the carotenoids combine with the oxidized portion of the photosynthetically split water molecule by forming epoxides across the numerous double bonds, with one or more epoxide groups resulting:

$$-C{=}C{-}C{=}C{-}C{=}C{-}$$

Such epoxide formation has been demonstrated in leaves and *in vitro*. Furthermore, our own recent studies have shown that when digitonin-extracts of *Euglena* chloroplasts are allowed to photo-reduce dye, an increase in optical density occurs at a carotenoid peak, 488 mμ. When transferred to the dark, this 488 mμ peak returns to the original level, indicating that the carotenoid changes can accompany the initial chlorophyll light reaction (24).

CO_2 Fixation

In a comparative study of the dark CO_2 fixation of microorganisms, Lynch and Calvin (81) found that *E. gracilis* differed from other organisms. Photosynthetic experiments of one and five minutes' exposure to radioactive CO_2 were performed. Not only were the characteristic dark CO_2 fixation products (malic, citric, aspartic, and glutamic acids) formed, but many of the phosphorylated compounds typical of CO_2 fixation in the light were observed. The majority of radioactivity, 84 per cent in one minute, 70 per cent in five minutes, was found in phosphorylated compounds. It was quite clear from their experiments that the coupling of energy made available by respiration and/or fermentation, with CO_2 reduction, existed in *Euglena* to an extent not found in any other plant or animal tissue examined. Further evidence of this close connection between dark and photosynthetic metabolic routes in *Euglena* was seen in the behavior of labeled acetate. Labeled acetate in *Euglena* in the dark found its way not only into tricarboxylic acid intermediates, but into all of the compounds usually found as intermediates of photosynthetic CO_2 assimilation. This is in contrast to the situation in *Scenedesmus*, in which acetate carbon in the dark finds its way only into the tricarboxylic acid intermediate. Assuming then that the mechanism for CO_2 incorporation in the dark includes metabolic pathways very similar to those used in the light, they represented the relationship between *Euglena* and green plant and animal cells, as indicated in Fig. 56.

The ability to utilize chemical energy for CO_2 fixation in a manner similar to that by which photochemical energy is used is limited to *Euglena*. Since *E. gracilis* is capable of carrying out all three types of metabolic sequence, in contrast to plant (as represented by the alga *Chlorella*) and animal (as represented by the microorganism *Tetrahymena*) cells, Lynch and Calvin speculate that *Euglena* represents a type in which the separation of the plant and animal kingdoms took place. They further suggest that the evolution toward the animal kingdom involved the loss of not only the photochemical apparatus but the ability to reduce CO_2 by the path of carbon-dioxide fixation.

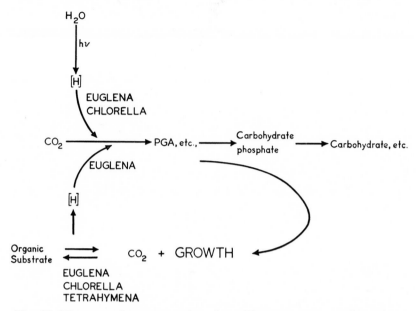

Fig. 56. Diagrammatic representation of possible enzymatic interrelationships among several organisms. Taken from Lynch and Calvin (81).

Respiration and Photosynthesis

Relatively little is known of the respiration of *Euglena*. Some species may occur at places where there is very little, if any, free oxygen available. The organisms may acquire oxygen by photosynthesis and are markedly aerotactic, but seem to be able to live during the dark periods in the complete absence of normal respiration. Measurements have been made of the respiratory activity of *E. gracilis* by Cramer and Myers (17) using Warburg techniques. They found that the endogenous rate for *Euglena* cultured photosynthetically was about 2.0 mm³ O_2 uptake/hour/mm³ cells. Determinations of photosynthetic quotients have generally been made with cells transferred from growing cultures to conditions of higher light intensity; the values available in the literature are all close to unity (31). For *E. gracilis* at high light intensities

$$Q_p = \frac{\Delta O_2}{-\Delta CO_2} = 1.085$$

We have measured photosynthesis and respiration by the Warburg technique in atypical gaseous atmospheres to enhance each of these processes in the absence of the other. Photosynthesis was measured in a 5 per cent CO_2:95 per cent N_2 atmosphere with saturated chromous chloride solution in a center well to absorb O_2 formed. Respiration was measured in an atmosphere of air with 10 per cent potassium hydroxide in a center well for CO_2 absorption. All manometer experiments were conducted at 25°C; cells were freshly harvested, washed once, and resuspended in 0.3003 M KH_2PO_4 at pH 4.5. The results are expressed in terms of P_Q/R_Q, where P_Q is the number of μl of CO_2 uptake per hour under the photosynthetic conditions, and R_Q is the number of μl of O_2 uptake per hour under the respiratory conditions. The chlorophyll concentration was determined for comparison with the relative P_Q/R_Q values. It will be noted in Table 20 and, more

TABLE 20

PHOTOSYNTHETIC AND RESPIRATORY DATA FOR *E. gracilis*

Experiment description	Chlorophyll conc. mg/ml $\times 10^4$	$-CO_2/+O_2$ in $\mu l/hr$	P_Q/R_Q
Light-grown	537.1	238/6.0	39.7
"Heat-treated"	<0.1	6.3/8.9	0.71
Dark-grown	<0.1	4.5/49.2	0.09
Dark-grown → light-grown			
1 hour	8.79	4.9/39.9	0.12
1 day	20.94	31.4/7.8	4.0
2 days	52.94	37.7/4.95	13.1
3 days	179.17	68.2/1.6	42.5

graphically, in Fig. 57, that in the light-grown organisms the P_Q/R_Q ratio was found to be around 40; in the dark-grown organisms, measured in darkness, a very low ratio of less than 0.1 was obtained. The photosynthetic uptake for *E. gracilis* at light-saturation was 130 μl CO_2/hour/g at 25°C, whereas at one-half light-saturation it was 90 μl CO_2/hour/g. The respiratory uptake for dark-grown *E. gracilis* at 25°C was 75 μl/hour/g.

The relative effectiveness of different wavelengths to induce photosynthetic activity was determined by measuring the oxygen evolution and carbon dioxide uptake of light-grown organisms. Carbon dioxide

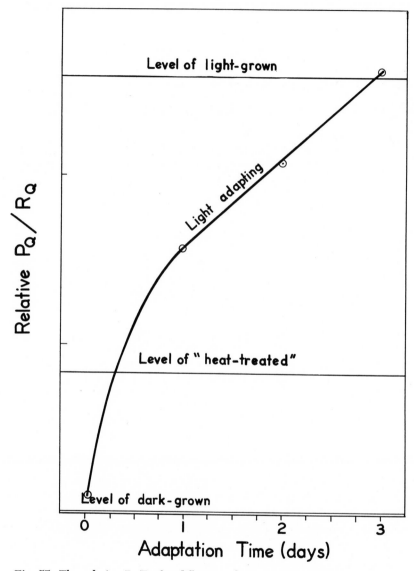

Fig. 57. The relative P_Q/R_Q for different cultures of *E. gracilis* during adaptation.

was measured in an experiment using chromous chloride to absorb oxygen; oxygen was determined in a subsequent experiment, without any gas absorbent, by the difference between carbon dioxide uptake and total assimilatory gas exchange. Both types of measurement were made in a nitrogen-carbon dioxide atmosphere. No correction was made for a small amount of respiration. The results of these experiments are given in Table 21 and shown graphically in Fig. 58. One

TABLE 21

RELATIVE EFFECTIVENESS OF DIFFERENT WAVELENGTHS
FOR THE INDUCTION OF PHOTOSYNTHETIC ACTIVITY *

Dominant wavelength, $m\mu$	$+O_2$ $\mu l/hour$	$-CO_2$ $\mu l/hour$
420	74.0	35.5
437	29.5	39.6
462	6.5	14.8
480	13.2	1.5
545	4.0	7.0
586	6.3	5.6
610	13.1	14.9
630	36.0	63.2
667	27.5	36.0

* All values corrected for light source emission, relative intensities, and number of einsteins per quantum.

would expect that these two curves would be similar. The results of these experiments indicate that red light at 630 $m\mu$ appears to be more effective than a wavelength closer to the chlorophyll absorption maximum in the red, 667 $m\mu$, used in these experiments. This is indicated for both the Hill reaction and for the total photosynthetic process. In addition, the Hill reaction or oxygen-evolving reaction does not show a maximum at 437 $m\mu$, which one would expect if chlorophyll were the only pigment responsible for light absorption; but rather, it shows greater activity further in the blue at 420 $m\mu$.

The wavelengths most effective for both chlorophyll synthesis and photosynthesis during light-adaptation resemble those for chlorophyll

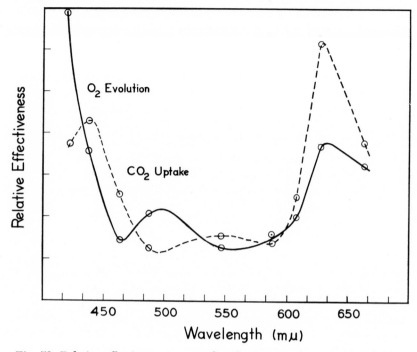

Fig. 58. Relative effectiveness vs. wavelength; CO_2 uptake and O_2 evolution, for photosynthetic activity.

absorption, with the possible addition of some other substance being influential for chlorophyll synthesis at 630 mμ. The greater effectiveness of 630 mμ than of wavelengths further in the red is less indicative of chlorophyll than of similar molecules. It is again suggestive that precursors are accumulated in low concentration in the dark; however, it has not been possible to demonstrate conclusively the presence of these precursors. Indications are that pigment synthesis and photosynthesis are not directly dependent on the same factors during the early stages of light adaptation. After 24 hours, however, both of these processes become linear, indicating that in the later phase of adaptation the two processes are dependent on the same limiting conditions.

Photochemical Activity of the Pigment-Complex

Digitonin is used to extract the photosensitive visual pigment-complex, rhodopsin, from the retinal rods of the eye. When rhodopsin is extracted, a light-dependent reaction, analogous to that occurring in the intact retina, can be measured spectrophotometrically. This photochemical reaction "bleaches" rhodopsin to lumirhodopsin; this is accompanied by a shift of the absorption peak from 500 mμ to 385 mμ (158, 159). The pigment-complex, chloroplastin, extracted by digitonin from the chloroplasts of *Euglena*, shows no similar shift in spectra as observed with rhodopsin. Chloroplastin bleaches at a rate proportional to the total amount of photo and thermal energy absorbed, causing a steady decrease in optical density with the disappearance of the maximum absorption chlorophyll peak at 675 mμ. Chlorophyll is bleached to unknown products. The spectral changes in the bleaching of rhodopsin and chloroplastin are noted in Fig. 59.

The most direct method of measuring the primary photochemical reaction is to observe the rate of photoreduction of the dye 2,6, dichlorobenzenoneindophenol at 600 mμ in the spectrophotometer. During photosynthesis, water-splitting reduction provides the chemical-reducing power which is trapped by the dye, and consequently, the dye is reduced to a colorless form. A second method determines the oxygen-evolving power and is referred to as the Hill reaction, in which molecular oxygen is produced photosynthetically. Thirdly, there is a method that measures the conversion of inorganic phosphate to biological high-energy phosphate. Adenosine triphosphate (ATP), the high-energy compound, is presumably the first stable chemical compound which can be isolated that contains the energy derived from light. ATP production and inorganic phosphate disappearance are chemically followed during the reaction.

These steps were followed through as a test for the photochemical activity for chloroplastin: The rate of photoreduction of the dye 2,6-dichlorobenzenoneindophenol (3×10^{-5} M) was measured at 600 mμ after illumination from one to four minutes with 300 foot candles at 25°C, pH of 7.0 ± 0.1 (in 0.1 M phosphate buffer). In 20 per cent of the preparations, photoreduction of the dye was complete within two minutes, with no accompanying reduction in darkness. In those extracts that exhibited active dye-reduction, an absorption peak at 488 mμ, that of one of the *Euglena* carotenoids, increased in the light and then decreased in the dark to its original level. The reaction can be repeated several times by placing the reactants alternately in light and darkness, without further addition of dye. This indicates that there is an increase in the amount of carotenoid absorbing at 488 mμ simultaneously with the dye reduction. Nieman and Vennesland (96) demonstrated a cytochrome *c* photo-oxidase in digitonin extracts of higher plant chloroplasts. Extracts yielding active photoreduction of dye were

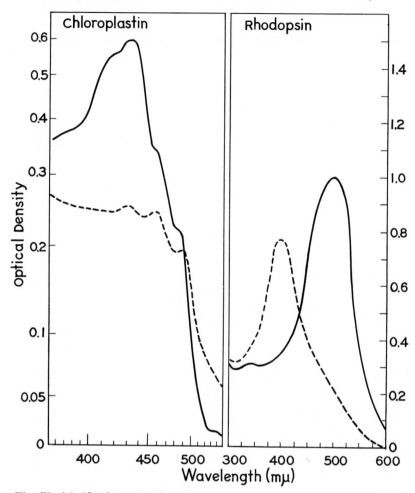

Fig. 59. (a) Bleaching of chloroplastin in white light at 25°C. Extract prepared from light-grown *Euglena* in 1.8 per cent digitonin, pH 7.2 (———— 0 hours; ------ 24 hours). (b) Bleaching of rhodopsin according to Wald (158, 159).

tested for their ability to cause photolysis or evolution of oxygen. Photolysis was measured manometrically in completely anaerobic Warburg vessels with KOH in the center well. The reaction conditions were the same as for dye reduction, except that the system for photolysis measurements was made oxygen-free to permit a qualitative identification of oxygen evolved by bacterial bioluminescence. Photolysis occurred with yields of 20 to 30 μl of O_2 in two minutes. This showed a distinct luminescent glow persisting for a minute after an anaerobic suspension of *Photobacterium phosphoreum* (in 3 per cent NaCl-phosphate buffer) was injected into the system in darkness.

In the experiments in which photolysis occurred, a light-catalyzed conversion of inorganic phosphate into labile phosphate was observed over a one-hour period in a similar anaerobic system containing six cofactors and adenosine monophosphate. The reaction vessels contained 2 ml of chloroplastin (having a chlorophyll concentration of about 10^{-5} M), 20 μM of Mg^{++}, 30 μM of alpha keto-glutarate, 0.3 μM of riboflavin-5-phosphate, 0.6 μM of menadione (vitamin K_3), 2 μM of ascorbate, 5 μg of cytochrome c, 55 μM of adenosine monophosphate, and 4 μg of inorganic phosphate; inorganic and labile phosphate were measured by Fiske and Subbarow (30) and by Crane and Lipmann (18) techniques. In one case, 700 μg of inorganic phosphate disappeared, but only 180 μg of labile phosphate could be found; in another, 550 μg of inorganic phosphate disappeared and 200 μg of labile phosphate was found. These experiments were immediately repeated with the addition of glucose and hexokinase, and the glucose-6-phosphate formed was determined by triphospho-pyridine nucleotide reduction at 340 mμ in the presence of glucose-6-phosphate dehydrogenase. In this way 80 to 90 per cent of the inorganic phosphate that disappeared was accounted for as labile phosphate. The phosphate conversion occurring in dark controls was only 3 to 4 per cent of that found in the light. Whether all of the cofactors play a role in the reaction is as yet unknown. These results, however, do indicate that some typical photosynthetic reactions can be observed with *Euglena* chloroplastin, and give some promise of being able, under the right conditions, to reproduce some of the primary steps of photosynthesis outside of the living cell.

Cytochromes

Before concluding this discussion on photosynthesis, I would like to say something more on the photochemical activity of chloroplastin and its relation to the heme-proteins, the cytochromes, in *Euglena*.

Recent findings suggest that a photosynthetic enzyme, a cytochrome or a cytochrome system, is coupled to the photoactive pigment-protein complex of the chloroplast, in which the initial products of the photochemical process function as H-donors and H-acceptors in electron transfer through cytochromes (5, 68). Such cytochromes designated as cytochrome f, b_6, and modified c have been isolated from higher plants, algae, and photosynthetic bacteria (5, 19, 54, 68, 97). Furthermore, there is the possibility that the photochemistry initiated by light absorption involves the cytochromes directly (15). (See p. 123.)

The question, then, is whether the photochemical activity observed for chloroplastin is also due to a cytochrome which is extracted by digitonin from the chloroplasts. In the experimental isolation of the cytochrome, the chloroplastin was precipitated with 80 per cent acetone in the cold. This precipitate was acetone-washed, air-dried, and dissolved in distilled water (pH 9.5). After standing, the insoluble proteins were centrifuged out and the water-soluble fraction was neutralized with dilute sulfuric acid. It was then fractionated in the cold with ammonium sulfate at 45 per cent saturation, and the precipitate was removed by centrifugation. The brown supernatant was again fractionated with ammonium sulfate at 90 per cent saturation. The precipitate, now pink, was redissolved in distilled water, reprecipitated with 90 per cent ammonium sulfate, and dialyzed for at least 6 hours in the cold. The absorption spectrum showed that an oxidized form of a cytochrome had been isolated. The absorption spectra of the oxidized and reduced cytochrome from the light-grown *Euglena* are shown in Fig. 60. In the oxidized state, the absorption peaks are at 524, 412, and 355 mμ; in the reduced state, the absorption peaks are at 552, 523, 416, and 315 mμ. The cytochrome isolated is a *c*-type, as indicated from the pyridine and dicyanide hemochromogen (50a). These absorption maxima for the oxidized and reduced cytochrome resemble those of cytochrome *c* isolated from *Chromatium*, a photosynthetic bacterium (5, 68). They differ from those of the *Euglena* cytochrome 552 (97) and from cytochrome *f* (19, 54), in that the typical cytochrome *c* shift of the β-band fails to occur. The electrophoretic pattern shows three anode-migrating bands, a major slow-moving band containing the cytochrome, and two other rapidly migrating bands. Cytochrome *f* also moves toward the anode, while the *c*-type cytochrome from photosynthetic bacteria and the *Euglena* cytochrome 552 move toward the cathode. The ratio of chlorophyll to cytochrome was found to be 300:1, in agreement with the chlorophyll to cytochrome *f* ratio obtained by Hill and his coworkers.

A cytochrome was similarly isolated in the oxidized state from dark-grown *Euglena*, and had absorption peaks at 530 and 412 mμ; when reduced, the peaks were at 556, 525, and 412 mμ (Fig. 61). The spectrum, however, is not that of a typical cytochrome *c*. It is closer to the spectrum of cytochrome *f* and a modified *c*, which are peculiar to the photosynthetic cells; however, as indicated, dark-grown *Euglena*

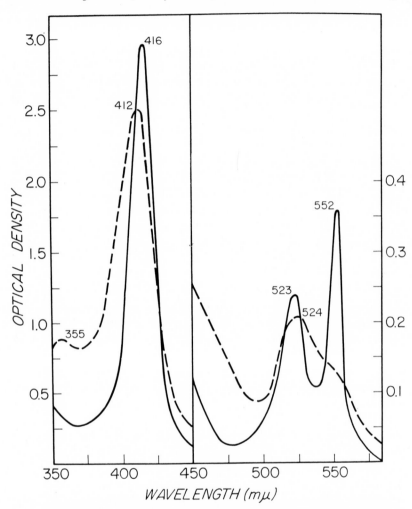

Fig. 60. Absorption spectra of the cytochrome isolated from the digitonin-extract of photosynthetic light-grown *Euglena*. The solid line (———) is the spectrum of the reduced cytochrome; the broken line (---) is the spectrum of the oxidized cytochrome.

are not photosynthetic, but resume chlorophyll synthesis and photosynthesis in a matter of hours when returned to light. This (dark) cytochrome may be part of the respiratory electron-transport mechanism. If so, this cytochrome should also be present in the photosynthetic organisms, but its spectrum could be masked due to its low concentration.

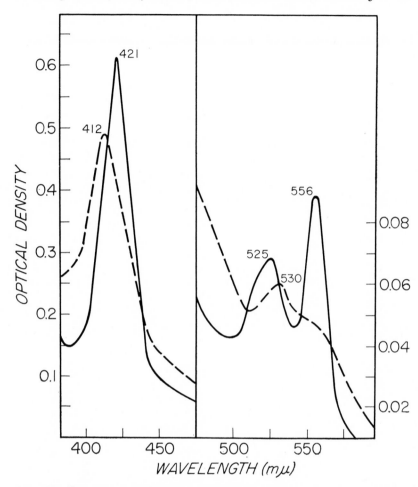

Fig. 61. Absorption spectra of the cytochrome isolated from the digitonin-extract of non-photosynthetic dark-grown *Euglena*. The solid line (———) is the spectrum of the reduced cytochromes; the broken line (- - -) is the spectrum of the oxidized cytochrome.

At different times during the dark ⟶ light adaptation, these cytochromes were isolated. In the first 24 hours, when euglenas are actively synthesizing chlorophyll, only the dark-grown cytochrome-556 could be isolated; however, when one complete generation time in the light has elapsed and the euglenas are actively photosynthesizing, cytochrome-552 is then found. The concentration of cytochrome-552 is directly dependent on chlorophyll synthesis until a constant ratio

TABLE 22

COMPARITIVE PROPERTIES OF SOME C-TYPE CYTOCHROMES

Properties	Algal cytochrome c, E. gracilis (50a, 97)			Bacterial cytochrome c (5, 68, 68a)		Higher plant cytochrome f (68, 68a)	Beef heart cytochrome c (68, 68a)
	Digitonin-extract		Acid-extract	R. rubrum	Chromatium		
	light-grown	dark-grown	light-grown				
Absorption maximum (mμ)							
Oxidized α	524	530	530	535	525	535	535
γ	412	412	411	409	410	412	410
Reduced α	552	556	552	550	552	555	550
β	523	525	523	521	523	526	521
γ	416	421	417	416	416	417	416
Isoelectric point (pH)	5.0	<7.0	—	7.0	5.4	4.7	10.0
Electrophoretic mobility pH 7 (cm^2/volt-sec) x 10^5	−7.9	—	+6.0	+3.1	+6.3-8.4	—	+8.2
E$'_0$ in volts pH 7	+.35-.40	+.31-.33	+.36	+.32-.365	+.01-.04	+.365-.380	+.265
Sedimentation S$_{20}$	1.2	1.4	—	2.0	6.0	6.9	1.8
Molecular Weight	11,000 *	13,000 *	—	16,000	97,000	110,000	13,600

* Calculated from S$_{20}$ and cytochrome c (D,$\overline{V}$) data.

of one molecule of cytochrome-552 to 300 molecules of chlorophyll is reached, in about 96 hours. The similarities between the absorption spectra and other properties of this cytochrome and the plant cytochrome *f* and the bacterial cytochromes are compared in Table 22.

Further studies on the nature of these cytochromes, *i.e.,* their excitation states, are necessary in order to understand their functional role in the primary events of photosynthesis. (Arnon, D. I. (*Nature*, 134: 10, 1959, and *Scientific American*, 203:105, 1960) discusses the functional role of the chloroplast in converting light energy to chemical energy through an enzyme system in which the cytochromes are directly involved with chlorophyll in the primary events of photosynthesis.)

7   MOTOR RESPONSES

"If they think at all 'tis no higher
Than matter put in motion may aspire."
(J. Dryden, *The Hind and the Panther*)

The protozoan flagellates are the simplest organisms for the quantitative study of the relationship between stimulus and response. It is an attractive idea to see if there is a fundamental principle common to the movement of all organisms. Englemann (23) assumed that the rounding-up and crawling of an amoeba upon stimulation is the same in principle as the contraction of a muscle cell. Hill (53) regarded all animal movements as being generally related to one another. Most studies of cellular movement have been confined to the descriptive details of movements of protozoa, rather than being attempts to analyze the mechanism.

The responses of *Euglena* to light-stimulation of various durations, intensities, and wavelengths were experimentally determined. The eyespot (the photoreceptor) area of stimulation of *Euglena,* and the flagella, its locomotor system, have already been structurally described. The response to light is believed to be mediated by the light energy being absorbed by the pigments at the eyespot, which is then transferred to the effector structure, the flagellum.

It was noted that the flagella consist of a number of elementary fibrils or filaments (axonemata) embedded in a matrix and covered by a common membrane, not unlike nerve fiber. In addition, lash-like expansions (mastigonemata), or cilia, are observed around these flagella. The number of elementary filaments usually appears to be eleven; nine are peripherally located, while the other two are found as a pair in the center of the flagellum. Sometimes the central fibrils are missing. This general pattern of organization seems to prevail for all cilia and flagella of plant and animal cells.

The chemistry of the algal flagella that have been studied indicates that they are composed almost entirely of protein. This protein may prove to be similar to actomyosin, the contractile material in muscle. Physical and chemical studies of certain bacterial flagella have been made by Weibul (160). He was able to obtain appreciable quantities of flagella by violently shaking a suspension of young bacteria and subsequently purifying this flagellar material, which was indicated to be fairly homogeneous protein. On hydrolysis, this isolated protein yielded a mixture of the usual amino acids, but this protein differed significantly from muscle protein in that it was deficient in the sulfur-containing amino acid, cysteine. Some physiologists think that the contractile nature of muscle is in some way related to the presence of sulfhydryl (SH) groups. Preliminary studies of Astbury and Saha (3) by x-ray diffraction and infra-red spectroscopy indicate that the algal flagella may not belong to the same group of proteins as the bacterial flagella. The movement of flagella and the contraction of muscle appear to be kindred processes, however, since the mechanism may be controlled by a similar molecule, adenosine triphosphate (ATP). It has been calculated that the energy required for a single whip or contraction of a bacterial flagellum may require a few, or perhaps only a single ATP molecule (76).

It would be extremely interesting to know more of the physical and chemical nature of the algal flagella—matrix and sheath—and their relation to muscle, nerve structure, and excitation.

Photomotion

Euglena exhibits three types of motion: pulsating, sidewise rotation, and forward swimming. The forward swimming and the sidewise rotation are caused by the whipping motion of the flagellum at the anterior end of the organism. Photomotion is defined here for experimental reasons as *photokinesis,* the change in velocity or rate of swimming on illumination without regard to directed orientation of the organism, and *phototaxis,* the directed orientation of the organism to light of various wavelengths. The photokinetic and phototactic responses together are referred to as photomotion. Numerous investigators, particularly Jennings (65) and Mast (92), have studied the rate of movement of *Euglena* and other protozoa. It was found that the swim-

(a)

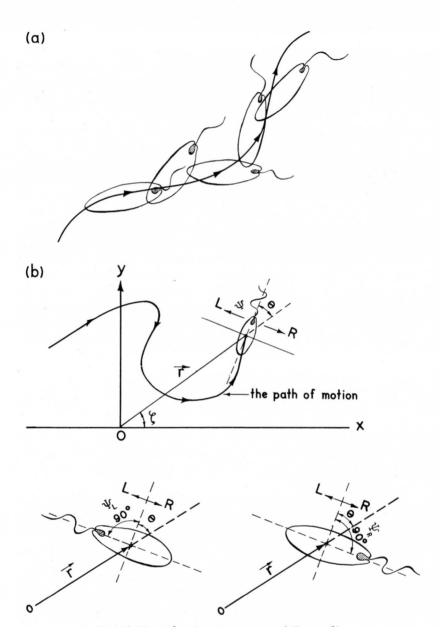

(b)

Fig. 62. Typical swimming patterns of *E. gracilis.*

ming rate of *Euglena* was dependent upon the absolute amount of light energy absorbed, that a constant rate of motion was observed at a constant light intensity, and that the rate of motion varied as the intensity was varied. Studies on the effect of pH and temperature on the rate of swimming have also been carried out by Lee (73, 74). However, there is still considerable controversy as to interpretation of the experimental results.

Photokinesis. The rate of swimming of *Euglena* was measured by suspending the organism in culture media which had a viscosity of 0.987 centipoises at 25°C. The measurements were made under a microscope in a dark room at 25°C by timing the distance an individual organism moved in a calibrated Levy counting chamber. The counting chamber was illuminated uniformly, and the intensity of light was controlled with a regulator. The light intensities were measured in foot candles with a photocell light meter on the surface of the cell chamber, and the meter readings corrected for sensitivity to the different wavelengths. A uniform distribution of illumination was maintained on the cell chamber through all the measurements. The velocity of free *forward swimming* without any *sidewise rotation* was measured by counting the number of squares on the chamber through which the organism swam and recording the time with a stop watch. A typical swimming pattern is shown in Fig. 62 (a and b). The average distance which *Euglena* travelled was found by plotting on graph paper the actual patterns of numerous organisms; to have statistical value, only those organisms which swam through fifteen or more squares were recorded.

Experiments were performed in white light, polarized white light, and for various wavelengths and intensities. For the experiments with various wavelengths, filter combinations were mounted at the light source, and the dominant wavelength of each filter was taken as the experimental wavelength. The relative energy distribution curves and the corresponding dominant wavelengths of each filter combination used are listed in Table 23. The light source was a General Electric 20 w daylight fluorescent tube, and the intensity was adjusted with neutral filters. It was observed that swimming velocity did not immediately change when a change in illumination was introduced to the organisms. It took 10 to 15 minutes for an observable regular pattern of motion to give symmetrical distribution curves. A lag period of 10 to 15 minutes for a change in velocity to take place following a change in illumination conditions was previously observed by Holmes (56) in *Volvox* and by Mast (92) in *Chlamydomonas, Euglena, Vol-*

TABLE 23

FILTER COMBINATIONS USED, THEIR DOMINANT WAVELENGTHS,
AND PERCENTAGE TRANSMISSION, TO MEASURE RATE OF SWIMMING

Filter combinations *	Dominant wavelength, mμ	Percentage transmission, %
5113 + 5120	418	11.0
3389 + 5113	442	5.80
3389 + 5562	462	38.0
3387 + 5562	480	26.0
3484 + 4303	545	15.00
2434 + 9780	600	18.0
2412	630	7.00
2434 + W-36	700	1.50

* Corning filter number. W, Wratten filter.

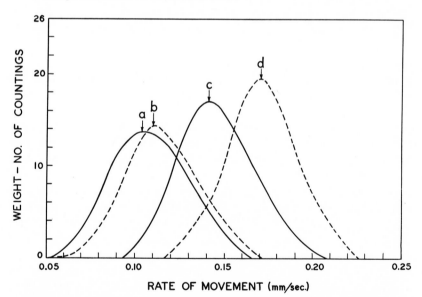

Fig. 63. The distributions of the swimming rate of *Euglena* in polarized and non-polarized light. Plotted weight, number of countings vs. velocity. The arrows indicate the centers of gravity. Note the shift of the peaks. (a) 4 foot–candles of white light, (b) 4 foot–candles of polarized white light, (c) 10 foot–candles of white light, (d) 7.5 foot–candles of polarized white light.

vox, and many other microorganisms. A possible interpretation of this reaction is that it seems to depend upon a mechanism that is only indirectly affected by illumination. A changed result with a change in the experimental conditions is defined as the degree of shift of the center of gravity of these curves (Fig. 63). It was necessary to make at least 80 measurements for each experimental condition for the data to fit a normal distribution curve.

The relationship between velocity and light intensity is shown in Fig. 64 (a). It will be noted that the mean velocity or rate of swim-

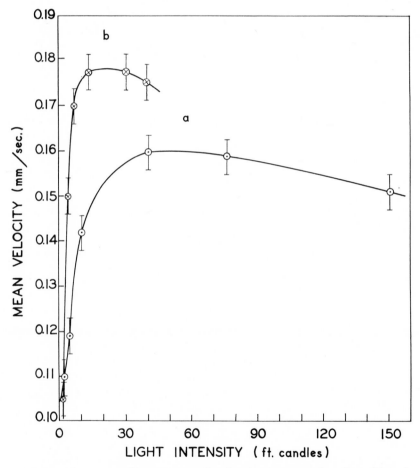

Fig. 64. The mean velocity or rate of swimming versus various intensities of polarized and non-polarized white light. (a) non-polarized white light; (b) polarized light

ming rises sharply from 0.11 mm/sec at 2 foot-candles until it reaches a maximum rate of 0.16 mm/sec at 40 foot-candles, the saturation intensity; it then starts to decrease slowly as the light intensity is raised above 40 foot-candles to 150 foot-candles. However, when the light is passed through a polarizer, the velocity steadily increases from 0.10 to 0.18 mm/sec at 13 foot-candles, and then remains constant to 30 foot-candles, as shown in Fig. 64 (b). The swimming rate in white light reaches a maximum average velocity of 0.16 mm/sec only when the intensity of light is raised to 40 foot-candles.

The significance of this value is that the number of light quanta at this particular intensity is sufficient to cover all the molecules which have a thermal energy equal to, or greater than, the minimal thermal energy, which is defined by the illumination and the absolute temperature. Beyond this intensity, the absorption rate will remain constant without being disturbed by the extra number of quanta falling on the molecules, since the maximum absorption capacity has already been reached.

The same effect was observed for various single wavelengths, although the saturation intensity was different in each case. The greater mean velocity of 0.18 mm/sec observed at 13 foot-candles of polarized light would indicate that polarized light is more efficient than is white light for this purpose.

In evaluating the relative effectiveness of various wavelengths on the rate of swimming, it was found that the mean velocity (in mm/sec) versus light intensity gave straight lines for light intensities of less than 15 foot candles. The action spectrum plotted for the rate of swimming (mean velocity in mm/sec versus wavelength at 4 foot candles of light intensity) is illustrated in Fig. 65. It will be observed that there is a major peak at 465 mμ and another peak near 630 mμ. The major peak at 465 mμ corresponds to a swimming rate of 0.18 mm/sec, whereas the peak in the red corresponds to a swimming rate of 0.16 mm/sec. This action spectrum is indicative of the absorption spectrum of the pigment involved in the rate of swimming. The peak at 465 mμ is suggestive of a carotenoid (perhaps β-carotene), whereas the peak at 630 mμ is suggestive of a porphyrin-like molecule (perhaps chlorophyll). The net effective light energy absorbed by the eyespot was calculated to be 1.7×10^{-11} ergs, with an assumed efficiency of 10 per cent. This calculation was made from our data, including the average cross-section of the eyespot (1×10^{-8} cm^2), the maximum

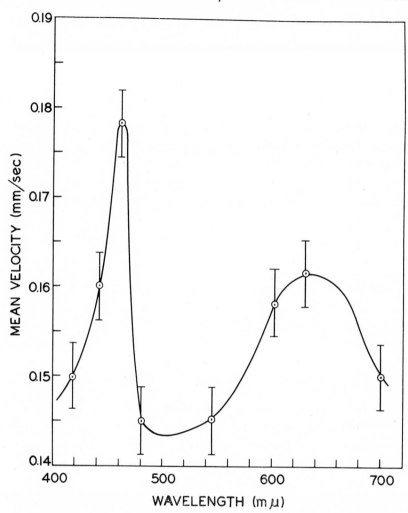

Fig. 65. Photokinesis action spectrum for the rate of swimming (measured at 4 foot–candles).

spectral accumulation peak at 465 mμ, and a light intensity of 3 foot candles (171). Lee (74) studied the forward swimming of *E. gracilis* from 6°C to above 30°C. The forward rate of swimming was found to increase with temperature, from 0.013 mm/sec at 6°C to a maximum of 0.08 mm/sec at 30°C. Above 30°C, forward swimming decreased to a rate of 0.038 mm/sec (Fig. 66). By comparison, the ciliated non-photosynthetic unicellular organism *Paramecium* and the flagellated photosynthetic alga *Volvox* swim at speeds of the order of 1 mm/sec. From Lee's experimental results, it is possible to calculate an approximate minimum molar energy of 66 k cal/mole or 4.2×10^{-11} ergs of light energy. It is interesting to note that these two methods of calculating the excitation energy are independent of one another, yet the calculated values are in agreement as to order of magnitude. This information could imply that the energy from the

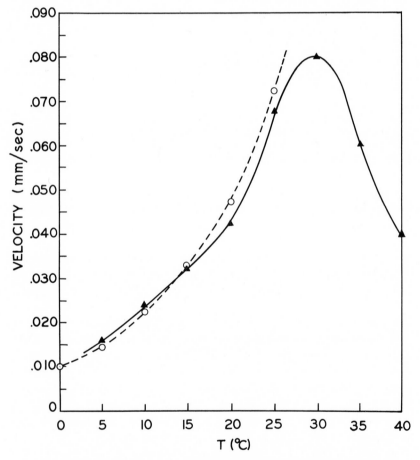

Fig. 66. Velocity in mm/sec vs. temperature for *E. gracilis*. Refer to Lee (74). (----- Calculated curve for increase in velocity with temperature.)

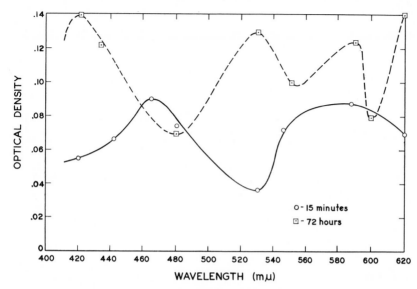

Fig. 67. Phototactic response to light of various wavelengths. Population density vs. wavelength.

light, if absorbed at the eyespot and transferred to the flagella, is sufficient to cause the whole organism to move.

Phototaxis. The degree to which *Euglena* responds more toward some wavelengths than to others can be studied experimentally by means of the phototactic spectral sensitivity, or action spectra. Bünning and Schneiderhöhn (12) recently studied the phototactic action spectrum for *Euglena*. However, many investigators over the past 100 years, including Loeb (77), Mast (92), Manten (89, 90), and Clayton (16), have studied phototaxis for *Euglena* and for many different microorganisms, without conclusive results. To obtain more information about the phototactic response of a population of *Euglena*, the organisms were dark-adapted and a known population was put into a long piece of glass tubing, in which various filter combinations were inserted along its length and adjusted for similar light intensities. The tube was shaken and the organisms permitted to swim freely in an area of their choice. Their accumulation in terms of density of population in front of each filter combination was determined at various time intervals. This is shown in Fig. 67, where it will be noted that after 15 minutes a greater density of organisms was found in a narrow region of 465 mμ and within a broader region of 570 to 600 mμ. The organisms were permitted to remain in the tube and to swim freely. After more than three generations' time (72 hours), it was noted that the organisms then accumulated at the wavelengths 420, 530, 590, and 620 mμ (close to the photosynthetic peaks), indicating that the absorbing molecules were most probably the porphyrins (chlorophyll).

For a more quantitative study of phototaxis, a simple spectrophotometer was constructed, as illustrated in Fig. 68. The apparatus is a completely enclosed black box, the only light that can enter the test

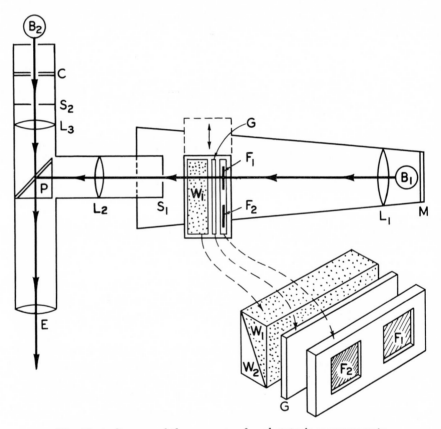

Fig. 68. A diagram of the apparatus for phototaxis measurements.

L₁, L₂, L₃—Convex lenses   E—Eyepiece
S₁ and S₂—Slits   F₁, F₂—Filters
B₁ and B₂—Light sources   G—Glass plates
W₁, W₂—Experimental   M—Mirror
          cell chamber   P—Half-reflecting mirror prism
C—Scale plate

cell is from the light source B_2. The light from the light source B_1 is collimated by the convex lens L_1 to the filter F. The glass plates G, are used to adjust the intensity of the filtered light passing through the experimental cell (W_1W_2). In the experiments, a suspension of euglenas was placed in the experimental cell compartment, W_1, and the culture medium in W_2 as a reference. The light that is transmitted through both W_1 and W_2 passes through the slit S_1, the lens L_2, and then is reflected by 90° at the half-reflecting prism P to the eyepiece E. W_2 counterbalances the deflection of the light passing through the prism formed by the organisms and medium inside W_1. The light from the light source B_2 passes through the scale plate C, then the slit S_2, and the lens L_3, and the scale is projected at the eyepiece where it can be read.

The principle upon which this measurement is based is shown by the equation:

$$\frac{I_0}{I} = Ae^{-kx}$$

where I_0 is the light intensity before entering W_1, I is the light intensity after passing a distance x through the suspension of organisms inside W_1, and k and A are constants characteristic of the organism and the medium.

Two filter combinations corresponding to two different dominant wavelengths, λ_1 and λ_2, can be placed simultaneously in the filter compartment, F, so that one-half of W_1 is illuminated with λ_1, and the other half with λ_2. If, at any instant, the concentration of organisms in W_1 on the side of λ_1 is greater than that on the side of λ_2, we will get a slit image shorter in vertical length on λ_1 than on λ_2. Then the relative spectral sensitivity for the wavelength λ_1 is defined to be greater than that for λ_2. By similar analogy, observations can be made for another filter combination corresponding to dominant wavelengths λ_2 and λ_3.

The advantage of using the wedge-shaped cell is that the light intensity transmitted is a negative exponential function of the concentration times the distance of transmission, and that the non-uniform vertical distribution of the concentration of the organisms is counterbalanced by making the angle of the wedge-shaped compartment W_1 sufficiently large. This makes it possible to obtain a sharper boundary at the top of the slit images. The effect of the different extinction coefficients at different wavelengths and the sedimentation during the observation were taken into account in the final evaluation of the experimental results. The limitation of the apparatus is that there is a certain upper limit in the intensity of the light source B_1. The light intensity for all experiments was kept constant at 15 foot candles.

The relative spectral sensitivities were determined for dark-grown, dark-adapted, and light-grown *Euglena* in both polarized and non-polarized light. In addition, the spectral sensitivity of *Rhodospirillum rubrum*, a photosynthetic bacterium, was determined (Fig. 69). The determination of this spectral sensitivity served not only as a test for the experimental design of the instrument, but as a comparative one

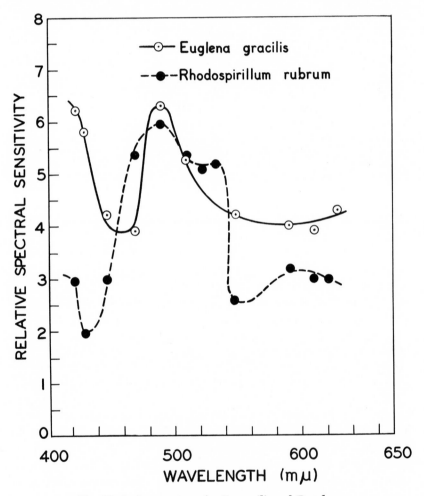

Fig. 69. Action spectrum for *E. gracilis* and *R. rubrum*.

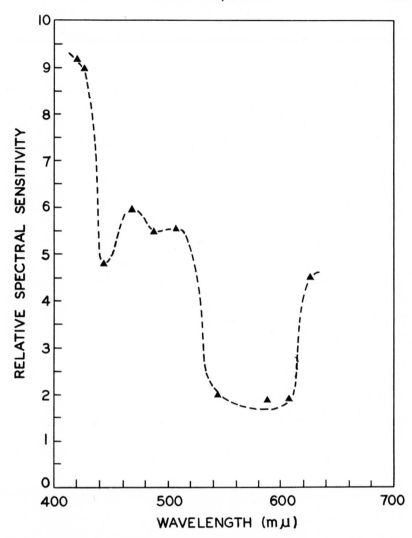

Fig. 70. Phototaxis action spectrum for light-grown *Euglena* in polarized light.

with the *Euglena*. The phototactic action spectrum for *R. rubrum* (7 days growth) showed peaks at 420, 465, 490, and 530 mμ, in general agreement with Manten (89) and Clayton (16). The action spectrum for light-grown *Euglena* shows a major peak at 490 mμ, with some sensitivity at 420 mμ, and with indications of a rise near 600 mμ. In polarized light (Fig. 70) there are maxima at 468 and 508 mμ. The maxima at 468 mμ and the one approaching 630 mμ almost correspond to the peaks of the photokinesis swimming action spectrum (Fig. 64). In dark-adapted and dark-grown *Euglena*, the maxima are at 490 mμ and near 600 mμ, respectively, very similar to the light-grown *Euglena*, indicating that similar pigments are responsible for light absorption.

The polarized light effects may be indicative that there could be at least two light-absorbing pigments. It has been suggested that β-carotene and/or astaxanthin are the eyespot pigments. If there are two pigments, the resulting polarized light effect could be due to a mutual energetic interference between them. According to Bünning's action spectra for positive phototaxis, a major peak in the neighborhood of 490 to 500 mμ and a minor peak in the neighborhood of 415 to 430 mμ were obtained; for negative phototaxis the major peak was at 415 mμ (11). The limit of sensitivity for both positive and negative phototaxis was at 550 mμ.

Our spectra are in general agreement with those of Bünning. However, we show that in addition there is some response beyond 600 mμ, but at present there is no explanation for the response in the near-red part of the spectrum. It may be the result of heat energy, energetic interference between two different pigments, or the presence of other light-absorbing molecules within the organism. Furthermore, we could be observing the phototactic response of *Euglena* at an intensity much lower than Bünning's minimum values of intensity required for any phototactic response. In *Tolypothrix*, a blue-green alga, Manten (90) indicated points of similarity with phototaxis in both flagellates and green algae. When the action spectrum of phototropism in *Tolypothrix* was compared with the absorption spectra of two isolated carotenoids from the organism, the absorption spectrum of β-carotene was in agreement with the action spectrum; therefore, he concluded that β-carotene acts as a sensitizer in phototropism. More recent studies on photoconductivity are indicative that β-carotene and similar C_{40} carotenoids can undergo cis-trans isomerization (as does retinene) and could well be part of the photoreceptor process (121). A comparison between these phototactic results and the eyespot absorption spectrum is illustrated in Fig. 71. It is evident that the eyespot absorption spectrum contains the same peaks as the complete *Euglena* action spectra. These data provide experimental evidence to indicate that selective absorption by the eyespot is linked to the photomotion of *Euglena*.

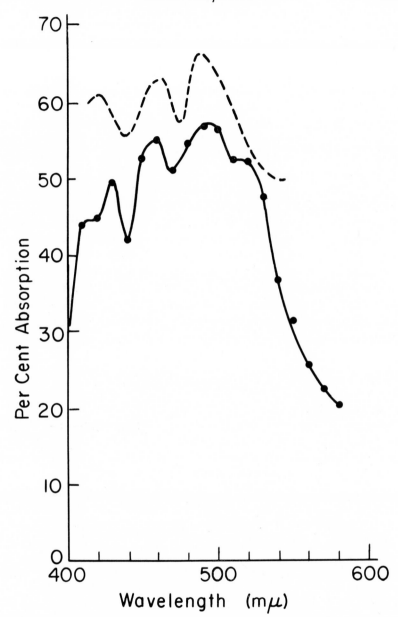

Fig. 71. Comparison between the phototactic action spectra (----) and the absorption spectrum of *E. gracilis* eyespot (———).

Eyespot + Flagellum

It is interesting to consider the connection between the eyespot and the flagellum as the most elementary nervous system. In *Euglena* the eyespot (the sense cell) is intimately connected with the flagellum (the conductor and the muscle-cell), linked so that light falling on the "eye" produces a movement. This structure is schematized in Fig. 72 and shown in the electron micrographs in Fig. 73. The translation of an internal effect into a surface action introduces problems similar to those involved in the origin of nervous impulses in animal photoreceptors. Clayton presents a strong argument for the similarity between phototaxis of *Rhodospirillum rubrum* and other organisms to the visual process in higher animals (16). Willmer suggests that structurally the most interesting features in the development of the retinal rods and cones are the flagellum-like fibers which connect the inner and outer segments of the retinal rods. He further speculates that embryologically the rods and cones arise from flagellum-like processes (163). The evidence of Sjöstrand (131-133), from electron microscopy, shows that the connecting fibers consist of a bundle of fibrils arranged in two connected rows not too unlike what is observed for the flagellar structure. Fauré-Frémiet and Rouiller (25) carried

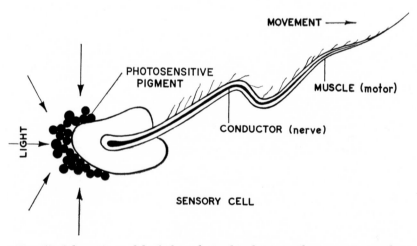

Fig. 72. Schematic model of the relationship between the eyespot granules and the flagellum.

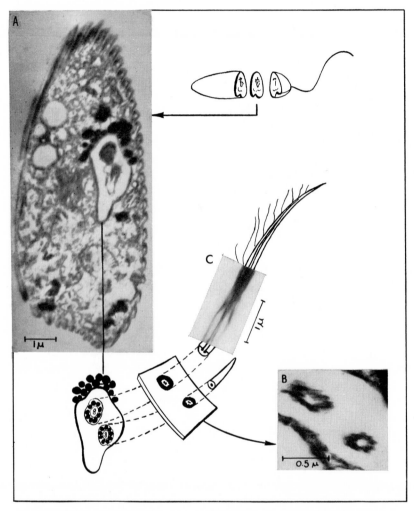

Fig. 73. Electron micrographs of the relationship between the eyespot and the flagella. (A) Cross-section of *E. gracilis*, showing orientation of eyespot. (B) Cross-section of flagellum. (C) Longitudinal section of flagellum.

this idea further and suggested from studies of the chrysomonad *Chromulina* that the second flagellum associated with the stigma possesses a fine (lamellar) structure similar to that of the outer segments of the vertebrate retinal rods and cones. If we are permitted to extend this point of view, we can look upon the *eyespot + flagellum* as really a "primitive eye" or the most "elementary nervous system."

From the area of the photoreceptor, the effective wavelength, and the light intensity, the energy necessary to produce a response can be roughly calculated. Castle (14), studying phototropism in the fungus *Phycomyces*, estimated from the area of the receptor and the light intensity that the energy is 1.9×10^{-7} ergs/cm^2/sec, assuming that 10 per cent of the radiation was absorbed. This estimation shows that the energy necessary to produce a perceptible mechanical response in the cell is small. The reaction time of *Phycomyces* under most favorable conditions is at least two minutes and may be as much as ten minutes. Delbrück and his associates are presently continuing this study with *Phycomyces* (20a). Our estimation for *Euglena* is 1.7×10^{-11} ergs, or a quantum efficiency of 14 per cent. The number of photons which can excite the "eye" at this frequency is seven. It is interesting to note that the human eye can detect a minimum of four photons at around 500 mμ.

The absorption spectrum of the eyespot implies that the velocity of swimming is proportional to the number of light quanta absorbed at the eyespot, and that the swimming motion is energetically controlled by light absorption at the eyespot. The shape of the intensity-dependence curve in Fig. 65, showing a gradual rise with increase in the intensity and the appearance of plateaus at higher intensity values, is very similar to the current-intensity curve of a photoconductive cell. It has been suggested that the creation of nerve impulses in visual processes may be considered as an event in which some electrical charge is produced by means of reactions derived from photo-activation of rhodopsin (122). The question of whether there really exists a characteristic threshold potential or not, and whether the energy transfer is done electrically, may be experimentally answered by measuring the potential drop between the eyespot and the flagellum; such measurements, however, are difficult to make.

In the photoreceptors of higher animals, the photoexcitation triggering the optic nerve, and for the most part the energy contained in a pulse, is derived from the chemical energy. Thus, the number of electronic charges involved in forming one such pulse is much larger than the minimum number of light quanta required to trigger the optic nerve. In the case of *Euglena*, however, such an amplification mechanism is not necessary. The minimum number of quanta required to excite the eyespot is comparable to the power involved in the swimming motion. This means that one light quantum which is effectively absorbed at the eyespot can be associated with approximately one electronic charge formed at the base of the flagellum. At the saturation intensity of about 40 foot-candles, the swimming velocity is about 0.018 cm/sec in a medium of viscosity 0.987 centipoises. Using the cross-section of the eyespot, the intensity of 40 foot-candles at wavelength 465 mμ (which is equivalent to about 2×10^{14} quanta per cm^2 per sec), and the average radius of the euglena, we have estimated the threshold potential to be of the order of 0.01–0.1 millivolts. This is small compared with the values found for nerves of higher animals.

The properties of the light-sensitive system in the bacterium *Rhodospirillum,* the fungus *Phycomyces,* and the protozoan *Euglena* appear essentially similar to those of animal photoreceptors, but the nature of their end-processes is of course very different.

Mechanism of Flagellar Motion

In *Euglena* and many of the colorless flagellates, the flagellum is attached at the anterior end of the body, and the cell is drawn along in some way by a sort of rotation of the tip. Lowndes (78, 79) made a study of the flagellar movement in certain microorganisms, and attributed the forward movement primarily to the oscillatory motion imparted to the cell by the flagellum rotating before it. The motion of the cell might be likened to that of a propeller with but a single vane, screwing itself through the water. Brown (7) was not content with any explanations, so he demonstrated the mechanism by constructing a mechanical device with a wire "flagellum" rotated by a twisted rubber-band. He also simulated a flagellated organism by himself; he submerged himself in a swimming pool, extended one arm stiffly in front of him, and by rotating it through a small angle, managed to progress at a speed of 10 cm per second or about four man-lengths a minute. More recently, a device similar to but more refined than Brown's was designed by Geoffry Taylor; it swam in a bath of glycerol, and the subsequent data and calculations emphasized the importance of the viscosity of the medium where the propulsion of microscopic forms is concerned.

The structure of the flagellum shows that there are eleven fibrils, two of which are in the center and surrounded by the other nine all wound in a helical pattern. The flagellum in *Euglena* is also made up of what might appear to be numerous conjunctions along its entire length. As illustrated in Figs. 72 and 73, the base of the flagellum is situated in the vacuole very close to the stigma (eyespot); however, it is not known whether the base of the flagellum is directly attached to the eyespot itself or whether the stimulation is carried from the light-absorbing pigment within the eyespot to the flagellum. In any event, this poses an extremely interesting problem for research.

Here we would like to add our own speculations as to the mechanism of the flagellum. The flagellum performs a kind of whipping motion very similar to that of a cowboy whipping his horse. The whipping reaction is probably adjusted so that the organism can move forward and backward or faster and slower. The light being absorbed by the pigment within the eyespot area would act as a continuous energy source for the motion. The energy flow is assumed to be non-continuous, but supplied to the flagellum in unit pulses. The fact that the motion of the flagellum is very smooth indicates that the total length of the flagellum, as a whole, forms a certain regular pattern. It is to be noted that one whipping is not caused by one single pulse, but is caused by the result of many small pulses being fired successively along a certain length of the flagellum.

Although no one has seen how the whipping causes the organism to perform with such a streamlined motion, it is suggested that the nine outside fibrils are perhaps wound helically around the two continuous central ones, although the electron micrographs do not indicate this. First, this was thought of as a simple propeller. In Fig. 74, the propeller is rotating clockwise, and the direction of the flow of the media is shown by arrows. Thus, the medium flows in the direction opposite to that of the motion of the beat of the propeller, either at the front or the tail of the organism. The surface of the propeller is so inclined that it pushes the medium to the back when it rotates clockwise, and forward when it rotates counterclockwise. If the nine fibrils were wound helically with a certain constant advancing angle, and the whipping were made by twisting the flagellum clockwise as in the case of the propeller, the medium in which the organism swims would be pushed backward. If the flagellum were twisted counterclockwise, the medium would be pushed forward. In the former case, the organism would move forward and in the latter, backward. The velocity would depend on the strength of the thrust, the number of whippings per unit time, and the distribution of impulse firings along the length of the flagellum. To keep the whipping action going at a constant rate, it is necessary that the thrusts should occur at certain intervals of length along the flagellum at a certain instant. Also, if a thrust is given at a point to the right, the next one should be given to the left to keep the motion at a constant whipping radius, instantaneously forming a circle. Therefore, it is conceivable that there is a

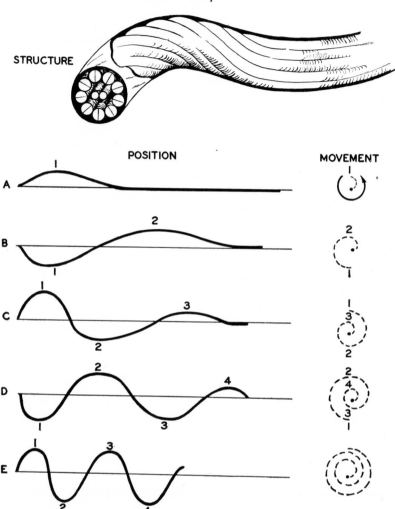

Fig. 74. Structure of the flagellum; packing of the fibrils that make up the flagellum. A, B, C, D, E—the whipping patterns of the flagellum.

certain feedback mechanism which lets the pulse firings occur at the side where the external mechanical stimulus is greater.

In the same analogy, the two central fibrils are thought to be energy-pulse carriers. One of them is designated the main pulse carrier and the other the feedback-pulse carrier. The nine outside fibrils fire the pulses at various junctions along the flagellum, while the central fibrils bring the pulses to the junction. The direction of the pulse transfer of the main pulse carrier is from the eyespot down to the flagellum, while the feedback-pulse carrier does it in the opposite direction. The latter and the nine outside fibrils are responsible for locating the right junctions at which to fire pulses. Thus, the feedback unit at a junction forms a feedback mechanism with the other outside fibrils. If a sudden shock is given to a point on the flagellum, it will cause a sudden reflective impulse at that point.

That the energy flow from the receptor to the effector is not continuous, but is in unit pulses, could be due to a certain threshold phenomenon associated with the photo- and electro-chemistry at the base of the flagellum, close to or at the eyespot. These are observed as successive trial-and-error movements in the course of hunting the place of optimum illumination. The sidewise oscillations or the gyrating motion of *Euglena* may be regarded as a part of the hunting process, similar to the rotating antenna of an anti-aircraft gun.

The fact that we can communicate with the organism by means of the intensity and wavelength of the light to such an extent that its speed and direction of motion can be controlled suggests that the organism may be regarded as a mechanical robot. These and other observations indicate that we may identify the eyespot + flagellum system with a kind of servo- or feedback-mechanism, or the most primitive form of central nervous system.

If we consider that the information received at the eyespot in terms of light quanta of various frequencies and intensities are converted into some other form of communication, and these new information codes are transmitted to the effector (flagellum) in such a way that the resulting responses of action are consistent with the initial information received at the eyespot, we can conceive of the following simple type of mechanism of transmission of information from the eyespot (photoreceptor) to the flagellum (effector) in *Euglena:* The information is transmitted by means of pulses of a constant height, where time of duration between two pulses defines the information being transmitted; each pulse carries a certain constant amount of energy so that the net amount of energy transmitted down to the flagellum per unit time is directly proportional to the number of pulses carried per unit time; a change in frequency of the light incident on the eye-spot brings a change in the time of duration between two pulses (the time interval decreases as the spectral effectiveness increases); a change in the intensity of light brings a change in the time of duration between two pulses; and, the information for selecting the direction of movement, or the "steering mechanism," is good enough only for selecting between two directions and no more, *i.e.*, between left (L) and right (R) in Fig. 62.

The rate of swimming and direction of *Euglena* can be practically controlled by external light conditions. This, then, permits us to conceive of a machine which may be able to perform exactly the same kind of motion as a *Euglena* on being illuminated by light. One possible machine of this type is a photocell schematically drawn in Fig. 75. In the diagram, P_1, P_2, and P_3 are photocells among which P_2 and P_3 are the phototactic receptors effective in determining the directional preferences, while the function of P_1 is to control the speed of motion resulting from the engine E and the propeller D. A_1, A_2, and A_3 are the proper amplifiers which will amplify the signals conveyed from P_1, P_2, and P_3 to B_1, B_2, and B_3, respectively. B_1, B_2, and B_3 are the devices through which the signals from P_1, P_2, and P_3, respectively, are observed as mechanical motion at D and C. It is supposed that the photosensitive pigment in P_1 has a characteristic spectrum like that of photokinesis (as shown in Fig. 65), while P_2 and P_3 contain a photosensitive pigment which has a characteristic effectiveness spectrum like that of phototaxis in Fig. 69.

Time-Clocks

The subject of phototactic responses cannot be completely discussed without referring to studies of "time-clocks." It has become evident that exact timing of reactions in organisms is of great importance. Many organisms show a rhythmic behavior pattern. Great numbers of lower organisms living in the seas have semi-lunar breeding cycles. Almost every species of animal is dependent upon the ability to carry out some activity at precisely the correct moment. In homing or migration, bees, ants, and birds use at least to some extent what is called "the light-compass reaction." They keep the sun at a fixed angle with respect to the long axis of the body. Other examples of physiological measurements of the course of time are provided by photoperiodic reactions in certain plants and animals.

The diurnal cycles of light and darkness are factors regulating endogenous periodicity. A change in the pattern of these external stimuli results in a shift in phase of the endogenous rhythm. When the plant or animal is raised under constant conditions, a single stimulus such as transition from continuous darkness to continuous light, or a short period of light interrupting continuous darkness, is necessary to evoke the periodicity.

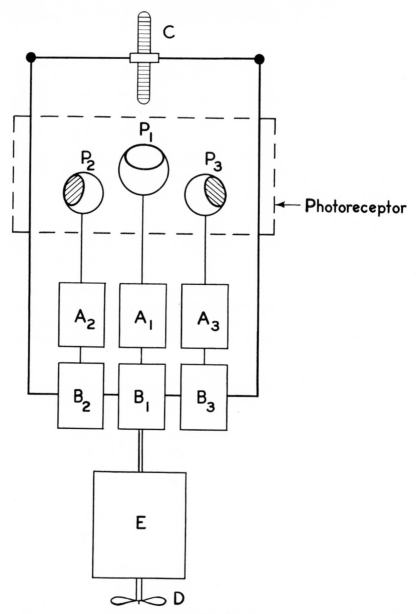

Fig. 75. Diagram of a photocell machine which may possibly be able to perform exactly the same kind of motion as *Euglena* on being illuminated by light.

This phenomenon can be easily studied with *E. gracilis*. Pittendrigh and Bruce (8, 9, 110) used a phototactic response; in their experimental procedure a narrow beam of light is passed through a suspension of euglenas. This beam of light acts as a "light trap" to attract the euglenas. It also serves as a sensing system to measure the number of organisms that have been attracted to the light, as well as the response time. The "test beam" is turned on for a short period of time, 30 minutes, at intervals of every two hours. This produces an endogenous diurnal rhythm in the phototactic response that is always very close to 24 hours and is temperature-independent in the range from 17 to 33°C. Pohl (111) also showed that *E. gracilis* has a similar endogenous rhythm.

Apparently, this can be best explained as a synchronizing effect on the stimuli of the several cellular "clocks." The external factors normally put the rhythm into periods of exactly 24 hours. The specific length of the period differs from day to day sometimes by only a few minutes, appears to be inherited, and is constant throughout many generations. Hastings and Sweeney (51) demonstrated a diurnal rhythm of luminescence which persists under conditions of constant low light and constant temperature in the unicellular dinoflagellate *Gonyaulax*, and suggested that these responses may be understood in terms of oscillating chemical systems. For a more extensive discussion of this phenomenon, reference is made to the work of Bünning (10, 11). The point to be made here is that there seems to be a common mechanism in biological "clocks" that can be more easily investigated with microorganisms. Here again, *Euglena* can be a useful experimental "animal" and one need not go into the complexity of the multicellular organization of higher animals to explore this phenomenon.

SUMMARY

"In spite of the attempt to collect from the literature all the information it offers,—It seemed more important to give assistance to future investigators than to devote much time to historical studies." (E. G. Pringsheim, *Contributions Towards a Monograph on the Genus Euglena,* 1956.)

Experimental studies have been described here that show how a microorganism, *Euglena,* can be shaped into a research tool for future investigators seeking answers to problems in morphology, growth, pigment synthesis, photosynthesis, photoexcitation, and other biological phenomena. The uniqueness of *Euglena* lies in the fact that it can greatly alter its chemistry and structure depending on its environment. These physical and chemical changes have been studied experimentally by microscopy, particularly electron microscopy, spectroscopy, and other analytical methods. The broader implications of these studies to the problems of light utilization by living systems, such as the structure of the chloroplast in photosynthesis and the eyespot and flagellum in photoexcitation, have been stressed.

The subtleties surrounding the question: is *Euglena* plant or animal? have not been labored. In light-grown euglenas, the chloroplasts suggest that it is a plant, but chlorophyll is not the sole criterion for being a "plant." The locomotion and movement of *Euglena,* controlled by means of its flagellum and by spiral movements between periods of "rounding-up" of its flexible non-rigid cell membrane, are animal characteristics. The "eye" and the "gullet" are also structural organs of the animal. The gullet is an aspect of euglena's structure which has been taken by some to indicate that euglena engulfs particulate matter, but no one has ever seen euglena eat anything. Taken together, these facts would indicate that *Euglena* in the light is a plant, able to carry on photosynthesis, but its behavior is that of a simple animal.

The region where a pigment strongly absorbs light will correspond to the wavelength of radiant energy which is most efficient in the promotion of chemical changes. Effective wavelengths of light of known energy were used to evaluate their efficiency in promoting a given photochemical reaction. By making appropriate measurements with wavebands throughout the spectrum, efficiency for pigment synthesis (or some function of the reaction) was plotted against wavelength to obtain an idea of the absorption spectrum of the pigment involved in the reaction. This technique of obtaining action or efficiency spectra has been utilized to relate a pigment to a process and to discover pigments not detectable by other means.

In general, it was found that the light-dependency for pigment formation in *Euglena* is not unlike that for the "greening" of some higher plants which are pale or etiolated in the dark. Etiolated plants contain a very faint "green" pigment (protochlorophyll). Protochlorophyll differs from chlorophyll by the absence of two hydrogen atoms. Frank, by determining the efficiency of various wavelengths, demonstrated that light which was most effective for the production of chlorophyll in seedlings coincides with the spectrum of protochlorophyll (33). Here protochlorophyll acts as a "trigger substance" to absorb light for chlorophyll synthesis. This was thought to be the clue to euglena's mechanism of synthesizing chlorophyll and building chloroplasts. Indeed, in chlorophyll synthesis the efficiency spectrum for "greening" in *Euglena* is very similar to that of higher plants. But there are at least two differences: firstly, there is usually a lag phase at the onset of synthesis which is not present in some higher plants; and, secondly, it is difficult to isolate protochlorophyll from the dark-grown *Euglena*. The fact that very few molecules of protochlorophyll and necessary enzymes are present in the dark-grown organisms suggests that other precursors may be present. Protochlorophyll could well be the light acceptor, but another compound, such as magnesium vinyl pheoporphyrin a_5, could be one of these dark-accumulated precursor molecules.

Porphyrins have been extracted from light-adapted, dark-grown, and a chlorophyll-free mutant of *Euglena*. The action spectra for chlorophyll and carotenoid synthesis have been shown to almost coincide, indicating that a similar porphyrin-like molecule may influence the synthesis of both pigments (167). It has been postulated that a photosynthetic enzyme, a cytochrome (an iron-porphyrin), is intimately linked with oxidation-reduction in the chloroplast and is part of the primary events of photosynthesis. A cytochrome, c-type, which is similar to the cytochrome c isolated from photosynthetic bacteria, was isolated from the light-grown *Euglena*. However, a c-type cytochrome was also isolated from dark-grown *Euglena,* and was similar to the cytochrome f isolated from the chloroplasts of higher plants. These experimental results suggest then that such a system or several compounds in the biosynthetic sequence could transfer their energy from one molecule to other pigment molecules in initiating photosynthesis.

After chlorophyll synthesis starts, chlorophyll rapidly increases and then keeps pace with cell division; chlorophyll per cell remains constant. This mechanism is no less mysterious than other examples of regulated synthesis. Why an organism stops growing is of no less interest than how it arises. This regulation is the essence of normal growth. Only so many chlorophyll molecules can be in a chloroplast. The tight packing suggests one mode of growth regulation on the level of cellular organelles. Does some critical volume ratio signal the end of chlorophyll synthesis? Obviously the converse could be the case; regulated molecular synthesis could determine organelle size. Perhaps the organelle size is further related to cell surface. It is striking that the number of chlorophyll molecules per chloroplast is a constant number, $\sim 1 \times 10^9$, for a variety of photosynthetic organisms, from microorganisms through higher plants (151).

The lamellar structure of the chloroplast of light-adapted photosynthetic *Euglena* strongly suggests that an ordered structure is necessary for chloroplast function in carrying on photosynthesis. The dense bands in the electron micrographs are most probably the "lipid-lipoprotein" layers; the pigments (chlorophyll and carotenoids) are believed to reside on the surfaces of these lamellae. The less dense structures are thought to be the aqueous protein layers. If the pigment molecules are spread as monolayers between the dense and less dense layers, the area occupied by the pigment molecule, determined from chloroplast geometry and the number of chlorophyll molecules per chloroplast, would provide a cross-sectional area of the order of 225 $Å^2$ available per chloroplast molecule. This is about the cross-section of the porphyrin molecule. If the chlorophyll lies as flat plates on the surface, then there would be a tightly packed monolayer of chlorophyll molecules spread on the surface with room left for only the necessary linear carotenoid molecules on each lamella. The lamellar chloroplast structure may be an efficiency mechanism rather than a critical functioning device. However, any forces, chemical or physical, that interfere with chlorophyll synthesis (such as removal of magnesium) disrupt the chloroplast structure. What we may have here, then, is a liquid-crystal type matrix which is necessary for the orientation of the active chlorophyll molecules.

In the dark, chlorophyll synthesis stops, and, as we have observed, the chloroplasts fragment. The organism makes no effort to rid itself of the remaining chlorophyll; it simply dilutes it out by growth. Under certain environmental conditions, poor nutrition, dark-adaptation, specific drug action, and temperatures above 33°C, a shift from chlorophyll to pheophytin occurs, *i.e.*, removal of magnesium from the chlorophyll molecule accompanied by structural changes of the chloroplast (164, 168). Pheophytin is perhaps utilized in other metabolic activities. Just where synthesis of chlorophyll does stop in dark-grown *Euglena,* and how far the chlorophyll molecule degrades, are difficult problems awaiting further research.

Other porphyrins present in *Euglena* are quite a few synthetic steps away from chlorophyll. They bear a closer resemblance to the pigment heme, the iron-containing porphyrin part of hemoglobin, than to known plant pigments. Chlorophyll is not free in the cells, it is bound to a large macromolecule. Is this chlorophyll-complex like hemoglobin, where the pigment heme is bound to globin? Because both heme and chlorophyll are porphyrins, it is highly speculative that we have in plants *chloroglobin* similar to animal *hemoglobin.* To learn something of the chlorophyll-complex in photosynthetic cells, the pigment-complex was extracted in nitrogen-free detergents such as digitonin and Nacconal; these pigment-extracts were identified as chloroplastin. Chloroplastin bleaches in light and heat, with an experimental activation energy of ~48 k cal/mole, similar to rhodopsin, the visual pigment. It was calculated from the analytical data that there is one pigment molecule per protein macromolecule, and that it has an average molecular weight of 20,000-40,000 depending on the method used to calculate the molecular weight. Chlorophyll combines with other proteins besides those in the plant; by complexing chlorophyll with other proteins, such as globulins, albumins, peptone, and gelatin, we have tried to learn something of the nature of these complexes (*i.e.*, the ratio of pigment to protein, the homogeneity, and the molecular size of the complex). The complex appears to combine preferentially with globulins rather than with the albumins. These complexes have some properties (physical and chemical) not too dissimilar from the native chlorophyll-complex in the chloroplast. The crucial test was to show that these complexes photoreduce a dye and evolve oxygen much as they would in the living plant, and this was demonstrated with some success with *Euglena* chloroplastin (24).

There are times when the organism's ability to make chlorophyll and chloroplasts, and hence to photosynthesize, is limited. Occasionally, a *Euglena* culture loses its ability to green. This is a sporadic event and so thought to be mutational. Within recent years, protozoologists have learned how to make *Euglena* lose its chlorophyll permanently by altering experimental conditions. Provasoli *et al.* (116, 117) noted that the antibiotic streptomycin inhibited chlorophyll synthesis. Pringsheim and Pringsheim (115) studied high temperature inhibition of chlorophyll synthesis, and later it was shown that an antihistaminic drug, pyribenzamine, did likewise (50b). These are permanent effects and the non-greening strains of *Euglena* thus produced never synthesized chlorophyll. This "bleaching," considered either as an induced mutation or, more narrowly, as a drug effect, is extremely interesting evolutionarily. Some theorists of evolution believe that an early stem "organism," with some photosynthetic apparatus, may at one point have been the progenitor of plants and animals, having gained an advantage over other simple living creatures in a world where organic food was scarce. Later, when plant life was well established and organic food plentiful, this type of creature may have undergone the same transformations we see in *Euglena,* losing its chlorophyll and becoming the first animal. Other theorists feel that *Euglena* is just one relic member of a large group of organisms, some colorless and others not, from which the plants, fungi, and animals evolved by separate routes.

We say, then, that in *Euglena,* the relation of the chloroplast to the organism is dynamic—and the organism survives without chloroplasts. It is a sort of *loose symbiosis,* not a tight one. Von Euler (156, 157) has tried to produce colorless maize by use of streptomycin. Before reaching sexual maturity, however, the plant died; perhaps here the relationship of photosynthesis and the rest of plant nutrition becomes too intricately interwoven to separate. As plant evolution proceeded, what may have originally been a chance association became a symbiosis, and finally a vital function.

Euglena has two flagella that arise from the bottom of the gullet, a rudimentary one and an active flagellum $\sim$30 μ in length. The flagellum is covered with a membrane and has lash-like cilia. The flagellum is constructed of eleven fibrils, nine of which are arranged on the periphery and two are in the center. This basic structural pattern of nine to eleven fibrils applies to all the cilia and flagella of plants and animals so far investigated. Additional chemical as well as physical research is needed to elucidate flagellar structure at a molecular level. The clues so obtained would be most helpful in the understanding of muscular contraction, nerve conduction, and excitation.

Light affects photomotion of *Euglena*. The rate of swimming increases to ~ 0.18 mm/sec with light intensity, until it reaches a saturation intensity. The spectral response curve for rate of swimming shows a maximum at 465 mμ and some response near 630 mμ; that of phototaxis shows a maximum at 490 mμ and responses near 420 and 630 mμ. With polarized light, the two response curves appear to be a combination of both the spectra for swimming and for phototaxis. The net external work done in photomotion is equal in order of magnitude to the light absorbed effectively at the eyespot. The eyespot spectrum shows that it absorbs light throughout the whole visible spectrum. There may be two dissimilar light-absorbing compounds within the eyespot of *Euglena*, β-carotene and astaxanthin, although the latter has not been isolated from the eyespot of green euglenas.

The eyespot and flagellum may act as the unit of phototactic responses. If so, one can think of them as structurally the most primitive of eyes or the most elementary of nervous systems, performing something analogous to reflex action. When dark-adapted euglenas were stimulated with light of a known wavelength and energy, the threshold energy necessary to produce the response was calculated to be about 3×10^{-11} ergs per whole eyespot. The human eye can detect a minimum of four photons at about 500 mμ; the *Euglena* eyespot a minimum of seven photons at 465 mμ. This corresponds to a quantum efficiency of about 14 per cent. The threshold intensity is about 2.7×10^{-3} ergs/cm^2/sec. Remembering that the eyespot and flagellum direct the dark-adapted *Euglena* towards the light for the synthesis of chlorophyll and chloroplasts, we see that the structures for locomotion, cited as characteristically animal, aid the organism in building its most plant-like attributes—the chloroplasts.

The question of whether *Euglena* is plant or animal is an "academic" one. By definition, a simple animal eats—the interest in *Euglena* is that it is related to organisms which are unmistakably animals, such as *Peranema*, but is perhaps very different from the animals giving rise to the metazoa. As we learn more about plants and animals, we see at the molecular level a common basis for all living processes.

We have tried to indicate how a "simple" organism can provide the research tools for many fundamental biological problems: growth, cellular structure, pigment synthesis, the relation of chloroplast structure to photosynthesis, and photoexcitation to vision. It becomes obvious that "simple" hardly applies to an organism that encompasses all these processes, each of which is still far from being understood.

APPENDIX

Media for Growth of Euglena

A. The medium for *Euglena gracilis* Z will serve for other highly heterotrophic strains of *E. gracilis*, such as var. *bacillaris*.

	g/l
K_3PO_4	0.20
DL-Malic acid	1.50
Glucose	10.00
$CaCO_3$	0.10
L-Glutamic acid	1.50
DL-Aspartic acid	1.50
Succinic acid	0.40
Glycine	1.00
Urea	1.00
Thiamine HCl (Vitamin B_1)	5.0×10^{-4}
Cyanocobalamin (Vitamin B_{12})	2.0×10^{-6}
$MgCO_3$	0.50
$MgSO_4 \cdot 7H_2O$	0.10
DL-Lactic acid	0.60
"Metals 47"	0.56

Metals 47	g/l
Zn as $Zn(SO_4)_2 \cdot 7H_2O$	2.64
Mn as $MnSO_4 \cdot H_2O$	1.24
Fe as $Fe(NH_4)_2(SO_4)_2 \cdot 6H_2O$	1.40
Co as $CoSO_4 \cdot 7H_2O$	0.24
Cu as $CuSO_4 \cdot 5H_2O$	0.04
Mo as $(NH_4)_6Mo_7O_{24} \cdot 4H_2O$	0.018
V as $Na_3VO_4 \cdot 16H_2O$	0.018
B as H_3BO_3	0.057

All the ingredients of this medium may be stored and dispensed as a dry mix, except for the lactic acid, which is added separately. For use, the approximate amount of distilled water is added, the ingredients are dissolved with the aid of gentle warming, and the medium sterilized as usual. One milliliter of the metals solution is added per 100 ml of medium. The pH of the final medium is 3.3-3.6 (See Hutner *et al.*, Anal. Chem. 30:849, 1958.)

B. For studies at alkaline pH's:

Medium 18	g/l
$K_2C_3H_7PO_6$	0.40
$MgSO_4 \cdot 7H_2O$	0.25
NH_2CH_2COOH	2.00
L-Asparagine	1.50
Sodium butyrate	1.00
$(NH_4)_6Mo_7O_{24} \cdot 4H_2O$	2.0×10^{-4}
$Na_3VO_4 \cdot 16H_2O$	4.0×10^{-5}
Nitriloacetic acid	0.10
Thiamine HCl (Vitamin B_1)	5.0×10^{-4}
Cyanocobalamin (Vitamin B_{12})	4.0×10^{-6}
"Metals 44"	0.28

One milliliter of metals solution per 100 ml of medium.

Metals 44	*g/l*
EDTA	2.5
$ZnSO_4 \cdot 7H_2O$	17.6
$MnSO_4 \cdot H_2O$	9.2
$CuSO_4 \cdot 5H_2O$	0.25
$Fe(NH_4)_6(SO_4)_2 \cdot 6H_2O$	0.70
H_3BO_3	0.57
$CoSO_4 \cdot 7H_2O$	0.04

Adjust pH with KOH. Check stability of pH by pressure cooking (KOH may contain much carbonate, which gives up CO_2 on autoclaving, with a rise in pH).

REFERENCES

1. Arnold, W. and Clayton, R. K. The first step in photosynthesis: evidence for its electronic nature. Proc. Natl. Acad. Sci. U.S. 46:769-776, 1960.
2. Arnon, D. I. Copper enzymes in isolated chloroplasts. Polyphenoloxidase in *Beta vulgaris*. Plant Physiol. 24:1-15, 1949.
3. Astbury, W. T. and Saha, N. N. Structure of algal flagella. Nature 171:280-283, 1953.
4. Baas Becking, L. G. M. and Hanson, E. A. Note on the mechanism of photosynthesis. Koninkl. Ned. Akad. Wetenschap. Proc. 40:752-755, 1937.
5. Bartsch, R. G. and Kamen, M. D. Isolation and properties of two soluble heme proteins in extracts of the photoanaerobe *Chromatium*. J. Biol. Chem. 235:825-831, 1960.
6. Bassham, J. A. and Calvin, M. The path of carbon in photosynthesis. Prentice-Hall, Inc., Englewood Cliffs, N. J., 1957.
7. Brown, H. P. On the structure and mechanics of the protozoan flagellum. Ohio J. Sci. 45:247-301, 1945.
8. Bruce, V. G. and Pittendrigh, C. S. Endogenous rhythms in insects and microorganisms. Am. Naturalist 91:179-195, 1957.
9. Bruce, V. G. and Pittendrigh, C. S. Temperature independence in a unicellular "clock." Proc. Natl. Acad. Sci. U.S. 42:676-682, 1956.
10. Bünning, E. Cellular clocks. Nature 181:1169-1171, 1958.
11. Bünning, E. Endogene Aktivitätsrhythmen. *In* Ruhland, W., ed. Handbuch der Pflanzenphysiologie. Springer-Verlag, Berlin, 1956, vol. 2, p. 878-907.
12. Bünning, E. and Schneiderhöhn, G. Über das Aktionsspektrum der phototaktischen Reaktionen von Euglena. Arch. Mikrobiol. 24:80-90, 1956.
13. Calvin, M. From microstructure to macrostructure and function. *In* The photochemical apparatus. Brookhaven Symp. Biol. No. 11:160-180, 1959.
14. Castle, E. S. Photic excitation and phototropism in single plant cells. Cold Spring Harbor Symp. Quant. Biol. 3:224-229, 1935.
15. Chance, B. and Olson, J. M. Primary metabolic events associated with photosynthesis. Arch. Biochem. Biophys. 88:54-58, 1960.

16. Clayton, R. K. Studies in the phototaxis of Rhodospirillum rubrum. I. Action spectrum, growth in green light, and Weber law adherence. Arch. Mikrobiol. 19:107-124, 1953.

17. Cramer, M. and Myers, J. Growth and photosynthetic characteristics of Euglena gracilis. Arch. Mikrobiol. 17:384-402, 1952.

18. Crane, R. K. and Lipmann, F. The effect of arsenate on aerobic phosphorylation. J. Biol. Chem. 201:235-243, 1953.

19. Davenport, H. E. and Hill, R. The preparation and some properties of cytochrome f. Proc. Roy. Soc. (London) 139B:327-345, 1952.

20. Davies, H. G., Wilkins, M. H. F., Chayen, J., and La Cour, L. F. The use of the interference microscope to determine dry mass in living cells and as a quantitative cytochemical method. Quart. J. Microscop. Sci. 95:271-304, 1954.

20a. Delbrück, M. and Reichardt, W. In Rudnick, D., ed. Cellular mechanisms in differentiation and growth. Princeton University Press, Princeton, N. J., 1956, p. 3-44.

21. Dobell, C. Antony van Leeuwenhoek and his "little animals." Harcourt, Brace and Company, New York, 1932.

22. Elbers, P. F., Minnaert, K., and Thomas, J. B. Submicroscopic structure of some chloroplasts. Acta Botan. Neerlandica 6:345-350, 1957.

23. Englemann, T. W. Ueber Licht- und Farbenperception niederster Organismen. Arch. Physiol. Pflüger's 29:387-400, 1882.

24. Eversole, R. A. and Wolken, J. J. Photochemical activity of digitonin extracts of chloroplasts. Science 127:1287-1288, 1958.

25. Fauré-Frémiet, E. and Rouiller, C. Le flagelle interne d'une Chrysomonadale: *Chromulina psammobia*. Compt. rend. 244:2655-2657, 1957.

26. Fawcett, D. W. and Porter, K. R. A study of the fine structure of ciliated epithelia. J. Morphol. 94:221-281, 1954.

27. Fawcett, D. W. and Porter, K. R. A study of the fine structure of ciliated epithelial cells with the electron microscope. Anat. Rec. 113:539, 1952.

28. Finkle, B. J. and Appleman, D. The effect of magnesium concentration on growth of Chlorella. Plant Physiol. 28:664-673, 1953.

29. Fischer, H. and Stern, A. Die chemie des Pyrolles. Akademische Verlag. M.B.H., Leipzig, 1940. Photolithographic ed. Edward Bros. Inc., Ann Arbor, 1943, v. 2, pt. 2, p. 55-58.

30. Fiske, C. H. and Subbarow, Y. The colorimetric determination of phosphorus. J. Biol. Chem. 66:375-400, 1925.

31. Fogg, G. E. The metabolism of algae. Methuen & Co., Ltd., London, 1953, p. 112.

32. Fox, D. L. Animal biochromes and structural colours. Cambridge University Press, Cambridge, 1953, p. 63-190.

33. Frank, S. R. The effectiveness of the spectrum in chlorophyll formation. J. Gen. Physiol. 29:157-179, 1946.

34. Frank S. R. The relation between carotenoid and chlorophyll pigments in *Avena* coleoptiles. Arch. Biochem. 30:52-61, 1951.

35. Frey-Wyssling, A. Macromolecules in cell structure. Harvard University Press, Cambridge, Mass., 1957, p. 61-63.

36. Fujimori, E. and Livingston, R. Interactions of chlorophyll in its triplet state with oxygen, carotene, etc. Nature 180:1036-1038, 1957.

37. Godnev, T. N. and Kalishevich, S. V. Chlorophyll concentration in chloroplasts of *Mnium medium*. Compt. rend. Acad. Sci. U.R.S.S. 27:832-833, 1940.

38. Goedheer, J. C. Orientation of the pigment molecules in the chloroplast. Biochim. Biophys. Acta 16:471-476, 1955.

39. Gojdics, M. The genus Euglena. Univ. Wisconsin Press, Madison, 1953.

40. Goodwin, T. W. Comparative biochemistry of carotenoids. Chapman and Hall, Ltd., London, 1952.

41. Goodwin, T. W. The biogenesis of carotenoids. J. Sci. Food Agr. 5:209-220, 1953.

42. Goodwin, T. W. and Gross, J. A. Carotenoid distribution in bleached substrains of *Euglena gracilis*. J. Protozool. 5:292-295, 1958.

43. Goodwin, T. W. and Jamikorn, M. Studies in carotenogenesis. Some observations on carotenoid synthesis in two varieties of *Euglena gracilis*. J. Protozool. 1:216-219, 1954.

44. Gössel, I. Über das Aktinosspektrum der phototaxis chlorophyllfreier Euglenen und über die Absorption des Augenflecks. Arch. Mikrobiol. 27:288-305, 1957.

45. Granick, S. Magnesium protoporphyrin as a precursor of chlorophyll in Chlorella. J. Biol. Chem. 175:333-342, 1948.

46. Granick, S. Magnesium vinyl pheoporphyrin a5, another intermediate in the biological synthesis of chlorophyll. J. Biol. Chem. 183:713-730, 1950.

47. Granick, S. Porphyrin biosynthesis in erythrocytes. I. Formation of δ-aminolevulinic acid in erythrocytes. J. Biol. Chem. 232:1101-1117, 1958.

48. Granick, S. and Mauzerall, D. Porphyrin biosynthesis in erythrocytes. II. Enzymes converting δ-aminolevulinic acid to coproporphyrinogen. J. Biol. Chem. 232:1119-1140, 1958.

49. Grell, K. G. Protozoologie. Springer-Verlag, Berlin, 1956.

50. Gross, J. A. A comparison of different criteria for determining the effects of antibiotics on *Tetrahymena pyriformis* E. J. Protozool. 2:42-47, 1955.

50a. Gross, J. A. and Wolken, J. J. Two c-type cytochromes from light- and dark-grown Euglena. Science 132:357-358, 1960.

50b. Gross, J. A., Jahn, T. L., and Bernstein, E. Effect of antihistamines on the pigments of green protista. J. Protozool. 2:71-75, 1955.

51. Hastings, J. and Sweeney, B. M. The mechanisms of temperature independence in a biological clock. Proc. Natl. Acad. Sci. U.S. 43:804-811, 1957.

52. Hedges, E. J. Liesegang ring and other periodic structures. Chapman and Hall, Ltd., London, 1932.

53. Hill, A. V. The laws of muscular motion. Proc. Roy. Soc. (London) 100B:87-108, 1926.

54. Hill, R. and Bendall, F. Function of the two cytochrome components in chloroplasts: a working hypothesis. Nature 186:136-137, 1960.

55. Hodge, A. J., McLean, J. D., and Mercer, F. V. Ultrastructure of the lamellae and grana in the chloroplasts of Zea mays L. J. Biophys. Biochem. Cytol. 1:605-614, 1955.

56. Holmes, S. J. Phototaxis in Volvox. Biol. Bull. 4:319-326, 1903.

57. Hubbard, R. The molecular weight of rhodopsin and the nature of the rhodopsin-digitonin complex. J. Gen. Physiol. 37:381-399, 1954.

58. Hutner, S. H., Bach, M. K., and Ross, G. I. M. A sugar-containing basal

medium for vitamin B_{12}-assay with Euglena; application to body fluids. J. Protozool. 3:101-112, 1956.

59. Hutner, S. H. and Provasoli, L. Comparative biochemistry of flagellates. *In* Hutner, S. H. and Lwoff, A., eds. Biochemistry and physiology of protozoa, v. 2. Academic Press, New York, 1955, p. 1-40.

60. Hutner, S. H. and Provasoli, L. The phytoflagellates. *In* Lwoff, A., ed. Biochemistry and physiology of protozoa. Academic Press, New York, 1951, v. 1, p. 27-128.

61. Jacobs, E. E., Vatter, A. E., and Holt, A. S. Crystalline chlorophyll and bacteriochlorophyll. Arch. Biochem. Biophys. 53:228-238, 1954.

62. Jahn, T. L. Euglenophyta. Quart. Rev. Biol. 21:246-267, 1946.

63. Jahn, T. L. Euglenophyta. *In* Smith, G. M., ed. Manual of phycology. Chronica Botanica Co., Waltham, Mass., 1951.

64. Jahn, T. L. and Jahn, F. F. How to know the protozoa. W. C. Brown Co., Dubuque, Iowa, 1949.

65. Jennings, H. S. Behavior of the lower organisms. Columbia University Press. Macmillan Co., New York, 1906.

66. Johnson, F. H., Eyring, H., and Polissar, M. J. The kinetic basis of molecular biology. John Wiley & Sons, Inc., New York, 1954, p. 272.

67. Johnson, L. P. and Jahn, T. L. Cause of the green-red color change in *Euglena rubra*. Physiol. Zool. 15:89-94, 1942.

68. Kamen, M. D. Hematin compounds in metabolism of photosynthetic tissues. *In* Gaebler, O. H., ed. Enzymes: units of biological structure and function. Academic Press, N. Y., 1956, p. 483.

68a. Kamen, M. D. *In* Allen, M. B., ed. Comparative biochemistry of photoreactive systems. Academic Press, New York, 1960, p. 323-327.

69. Karrer, P. and Jucker, E. Carotenoids. Elsevier Pub. Co., New York, 1950.

70. Kidder, G. W. Nutrition and metabolism of protozoa. Ann. Rev. Microbiol. 5:139-156, 1951.

71. Koski, V. M. and Smith, J. H. C. The isolation and spectral absorption properties of protochlorophyll from etiolated barley seedlings. J. Am. Chem. Soc. 70:3558-3562, 1948.

72. Krinsky, N. I. and Goldsmith, T. H. Carotenoids of *Euglena gracilis* (Z strain). Federation Proc. 19:329, 1960.

73. Lee, J. W. The effect of pH on forward swimming in Euglena and Chilomonas. Physiol. Zool. 27:272-275, 1954.

74. Lee, J. W. The effect of temperature on forward swimming in Euglena and Chilomonas. Physiol. Zool. 27:275-280, 1954.

75. Leedale, G. F. Mitosis and chromosome numbers in the Euglenineae (Flagellata). Nature 181:502-503, 1958.

76. Lewin, R. A. Flagella: variations and enigmas. New Biol. 19:27-47, 1955.

77. Loeb, J. Forced movements, tropism and animal conduct. J. B. Lippincott, Philadelphia, 1918.

78. Lowndes, A. G. The swimming of *Monas stigmatica* Pringsheim, *Peranama trichophorum* and *Volvox* sp. Proc. Zool. Soc. (London) 114A: 325-338, 1944.

79. Lowndes, A. G. The swimming of unicellular flagellate organisms. Proc. Zool. Soc. (London) 113A:99-107, 1944.

80. Lyman, H., Epstein, H. T., and Schiff, J. Ultraviolet inactivation and photo-

reactivation of chloroplast development in *Euglena* without cell death. J. Protozool. 6:264-265, 1959.

81. Lynch, V. H. and Calvin, M. CO_2 fixation by *Euglena*. Ann. N. Y. Acad. Sci. 56:890-900, 1953.

82. Lythgoe, R. S. and Quilliam, J. P. The thermal decomposition of visual purple. J. Physiol. 93:24-37, 1938.

83. Lwoff, A. Introduction to biochemistry of protozoa. *In* Lwoff, A., ed. Biochemistry and physiology of protozoa. Academic Press, N. Y., 1951, v. 1, p. 1-26.

84. Lwoff, A. L'evolution physiologique. Hermann et Cie, Paris, 1944.

85. Lwoff, A. Recherches biochimiques sur la nutrition des protozoaires; le pouvoir de synthèse. Masson et Cie, Paris, 1932.

86. Lwoff, A. and Dusi, H. La nutrition de l'Euglénien *Astasia chattoni*. Compt. rend. 202:248-250, 1936.

87. McDonald, E. Neutron radiation on living cells. Williams and Wilkins Co., Baltimore, 1947.

88. McKinney, G. Absorption of light by chlorophyll solutions. J. Biol. Chem. 140:315-322, 1941.

89. Manten, A. Phototaxis in the purple bacterium *Rhodospirillum rubrum* and the relation between phototaxis and photosynthesis. Antonie van Leeuwenhoek 14:65-86, 1948.

90. Manten, A. Phototaxis, phototropism and photosynthesis in purple bacteria and blue-green algae. Thesis, Drukkerij. Fa. Schotanus & Jens, Utrecht, Holland, 1948.

91. Manton, I. The fine structure of plant cilia. *In* Symp. Soc. Exptl. Biol. 6:306-319, 1952.

92. Mast, S. O. Light and the behavior of organisms. John Wiley and Sons, New York, 1911.

93. Mauzerall, D. and Granick, S. Porphyrin biosynthesis in erythrocytes. III. Uroporphyrinogen and its decarboxylase. J. Biol. Chem. 232:1141-1162, 1958.

94. Miller, G. L. and Andersson, K. J. I. Ultracentrifuge and diffusion studies on native and reduced insulin in Duponol solution. J. Biol. Chem. 144:475-486, 1942.

95. Myers, J. Physiology of the algae. Ann. Rev. Microbiol. 5:157-180, 1951.

96. Nieman, R. H. and Vennesland, B. Cytochrome c photooxidase of spinach chloroplasts. Science 125:353-354, 1957.

97. Nishimura, M. A new hematin compound isolated from *Euglena gracilis*. J. Biochem. 46:219-223, 1959.

98. Nishimura, M. and Huzisige, H. Studies on the chlorophyll formation in *Euglena gracilis* with special reference to the action spectrum of the process. J. Biochem. 46:225-234, 1959.

99. Noack, K. and Kiessling, W. Zur Entstehung des Chlorophylls und seiner Beziehung zum Blutfarbstoff. I. Mitteilung. Hoppe-Seyler's Z. physiol. Chem. 182:13-49, 1929.

100. Noack, K. and Kiessling, W. Zur Entstehung des Chlorophylls und seiner Beziehung zum Blutfarbstoff. II. Mitteilung. Hoppe-Seyler's Z. physiol. Chem. 193:97-137, 1930.

101. Palade, G. E. An electron microscope study of the mitochondrial structure. J. Histochem. Cytochem. 1:188-211, 1953.

102. Palade, G. E. A study of fixation for electron microscopy. J. Exptl. Med. 95:285-298, 1952.

103. Palade, G. E. The fine structure of mitochondria. Anat. Rec. 114:427-451, 1952.

104. Palade, G. E. The fixation of tissues for electron microscopy. Proc. Intern. Conf. Electron Microscopy, London, 1954, p. 129.

105. Palade, G. E. and Porter, K. R. Studies on the endoplasmic reticulum. I. Its identification in cells in situ. J. Exptl. Med. 100:641-656, 1954.

106. Palade, G. E. and Siekevitz, P. Liver microsomes. An integrated morphological and biochemical study. J. Biophys. Biochem. Cytol. 2:171-200, 1956.

107. Pease, D. C. Histological techniques for electron microscopy. Academic Press, New York, 1960.

108. Pitelka, D. R. and Schooley, C. N. Comparative morphology of some protistan flagella. Univ. California, Berkeley, 1955.

109. Pitelka, D. R. and Schooley, C. N. The fine structure of the flagellar apparatus in Trichonympha. J. Morphol. 102:199-246, 1958.

110. Pittendrigh, C. S. On temperature independence in the clock system controlling emergence time in Drosophila. Proc. Natl. Acad. Sci. U.S. 40:1018-1029, 1954.

111. Pohl, R. Tagesrhythmus im phototaktischen Verhalten der *Euglena gracilis*. Z. Naturforsch. 3b:367-374, 1948.

112. Porter, K. R. Observations on a submicroscopic basophilic component of cytoplasm. J. Exptl. Med. 97:727-750, 1953.

113. Pringsheim, E. G. Contributions toward a monograph of the genus Euglena. Nova Acta Leopoldina 18:125, 1956.

114. Pringsheim, E. G. and Hovasse, R. The loss of chromatophores in *Euglena gracilis*. New Phytologist 47:52-87, 1948.

115. Pringsheim, E. G. and Pringsheim, O. Experimental elimination of chromatophores and eye spot in *Euglena gracilis*. New Phytologist 51:65-76, 1952.

116. Provasoli, L., Hutner, S. H., and Pintner, I. J. Destruction of chloroplasts by streptomycin. Cold Spring Harbor Symp. Quant. Biol. 16:113-120, 1951.

117. Provasoli, L., Hutner, S. H. and Schatz, A. Streptomycin-induced chlorophyll-less races of *Euglena*. Proc. Soc. Exptl. Biol. Med. 69: 279-282, 1948.

118. Puck, T. T., Marcus, P. I., and Cieciura, S. J. Clonal growth of mammalian cells *in vitro*. Growth characteristics of colonies from single Hela cells with and without a "feeder" layer. J. Exptl. Med. 103:273-284, 1956.

119. Putnam, F. W. The interactions of proteins and synthetic detergents. Adv. Protein Chem. 4:79-122, 1948.

120. Rabinowitch, E. I. Photosynthesis and related processes. Interscience Publishers, Inc., New York, v. 1, 1946, v. 2 pt. 1, 1951, v. 2, pt. 2, 1956.

121. Rosenberg, B. Photoconduction and cis-trans isomerism in β-carotene. J. Chem. Phys. 31:238-246, 1959.

122. Rosenberg, B. Photoconductivity and the visual receptor processes. J. Opt. Soc. Am. 48:581, 1958.

123. Rudolph, H. Über die Einwirkung des farbingen Lichtes auf die Entstehung der Chloroplastenfarbstoffe. Planta 21:104-155, 1933.

124. Sager, R. The photochemical apparatus: Its structure and function. Brookhaven Symp. Biol. No. 11, 1959.

125. Sager, R. and Zalokar, M. Pigments and photosynthesis in a carotenoid-deficient mutant of *Chlamydomonas*. Nature 182:98-100, 1958.
126. St. George, R. C. Interplay of light and heat in bleaching rhodopsin. J. Gen. Physiol. 35:495-517, 1952.
126a. Schoenborn, H. W. Lethal effect of u.v. and X-radiation on the protozoan flagellate *Astasia longa*. Physiol. Zool. 26:312-319, 1953.
127. Schoenborn, H. W. Studies on the nutrition of colorless euglenoid flagellates. II. Growth of *Astasia* in an inorganic medium. Physiol. Zool. 19:430-442, 1946.
128. Seybold, A. and Egle, K. Lichtfeld und Blattfarbstoffe. II. Planta 28:87-123, 1938.
129. Seybold, A. and Egle, K. Zur Kenntis des Protochlorophylls II. Planta 29:119-128, 1939.
130. Shibata, K., Benson, A. A., and Calvin, M. The absorption spectra of suspensions of living microorganisms. Biochim. Biophys. Acta 15:461-470, 1954.
131. Sjöstrand, F. S. An electron microscope study of the retinal rods of the guinea pig eye. J. Cellular Comp. Physiol. 33:383-404, 1949.
132. Sjöstrand, F. S. The ultrastructure of the inner segments of the retinal rods of the guinea pig as revealed by the electron microscope. J. Cellular Comp. Physiol. 42:45-70, 1953.
133. Sjöstrand, F. S. The ultrastructure of the outer segments of rods and cones of the eye as revealed by the electron microscope. J. Cellular Comp. Physiol. 42:15-44, 1953.
134. Smith, E. L. The action of sodium dodecyl sulfate on the chlorophyll-protein compound of the spinach leaf. J. Gen. Physiol. 24:583-596, 1941.
135. Smith, E. L. The chlorophyll-protein compound of the green leaf. J. Gen. Physiol. 24:565-582, 1941.
136. Smith, E. L. and Pickels, E. G. Micelle formation in aqueous solutions of digitonin. Proc. Natl. Acad. Sci. U.S. 26:272-277, 1940.
137. Smith, E. L. and Pickels, E. G. The effect of detergents on the chlorophyll-protein compound of spinach as studied in the ultracentrifuge. J. Gen. Physiol. 24:753-764, 1941.
138. Smith, J. H. C. Protochlorophyll, precursor of chlorophyll. Arch. Biochem. 19:449-454, 1948.
138a. Smith, J. H. C. *In* Allen, M. B., ed. Comparative biochemistry of photoreactive systems. Academic Press, New York, 1960, p. 257-277.
139. Smith, J. H. C. and Kupke, D. W. Some properties of extracted protochlorophyll holochrome. Nature 178:751-752, 1956.
140. Smith, J. H. C. and Young, V. M. K. *In* Hollaender, A., ed. Radiation biology. McGraw–Hill Publishers, New York, 1956, p. 393-442.
141. Stanier, R. Y. Formation and function of the photosynthetic pigment system. The photochemical apparatus: its structure and function. Brookhaven Symp. Biol. No. 11, 1959.
142. Stern, K. H. The Liesegang phenomenon. Chem. Revs. 54:79-99, 1954.
143. Strain, H. H. Chloroplast pigments. Ann. Rev. Biochem. 13:591-610, 1944.
144. Strain, H. H. Indispensable leaf yellow. J. Chem. Ed. 23:262-267, 1946.
145. Strain, H. H. Leaf xanthophylls. Carnegie Inst. of Washington Publication No. 490, 1938.
146. Strain, H. H. Manual of phycology. Chronica Botanica, Waltham, Mass., 1951, p. 243-262.

147. Strother, G. K. and Wolken, J. J. A simplified microspectrophotometer. Science 130:1084-1088, 1959.

147a. Strother, G. K. and Wolken, J. J. Microspectrophotometry of *Euglena* chloroplast and eyespot. Nature 188:601-602, 1960.

148. Takashima, S. Chlorophyll-lipoprotein obtained in crystals. Nature 169:182-184, 1952.

149. The Photochemical Apparatus: Its structure and function. Brookhaven Symposia in Biology No. 11, 1959.

150. Thin-sectioning and associated techniques for electron microscopy. Ivan Sorvall, Inc., Norwalk, Conn., 1959.

151. Thomas, J. B. Chloroplast structure and function. Endeavour 17:156, 1958.

152. Thomas, J. B. The structure and function of the chloroplast. Prog. Biophys. 5:109-139, 1955.

153. Tischer, J. Über das Euglenarhodon und andere Carotinoide einer roten Euglene. (Carotinoide der Süsswasseralgen, I. Teil.) Hoppe-Seyler's Z. physiol. Chem. 239:257-269, 1936.

154. Van Niel, C. B. The bacterial photosyntheses and their importance for the general problem of photosynthesis. Adv. Enzymol. 1:263-328, 1941.

155. v. Euler, H., Bergman, B., and Hellström, H. Über das Verhaltnis von Chloroplastenzahl und Chlorophyll-konzentration bei Elodea densa. Ber. Deut. Botan. Ges. 52:458-462, 1934.

156. von Euler, H. Nukleinsäuren als Wuchsstoffe in Gegenwart von Colchicin und von Streptomycin. Arkiv Kemi Mineral. Geol. 25A(8):1-9, 1948.

157. von Euler, H. Einfluss von Streptomycin und Dihydro-streptomycin auf keimende Samen grüner Pflanzen. Hoppe-Seyler's Z. physiol. Chem. 295:411-413, 1953.

158. Wald, G. The biochemistry of visual excitation. *In* Gaebler, O. H., ed. Enzymes: units of biological structure and function. Academic Press, Inc., New York, 1956, p. 355-367.

159. Wald, G. The biochemistry of vision. Ann. Rev. Biochem. 22:497-526, 1953.

160. Weibul, C. Some analytical evidence for the purity of Proteus flagella protein. Acta Chem. Scand. 5:529-534, 1951.

161. Wichterman, R. Survival and other effects following x-radiation of the flagellate *Euglena gracilis*. Biol. Bull. 109:371, 1955.

162. Wichterman, R. and Honegger, C. M. Action of x-rays on the two common amoebas. Proc. Pa. Acad. Sci. 22:240-253, 1958.

163. Willmer, E. N. The physiology of vision. Ann. Rev. Physiol. 17:339-366, 1955.

164. Wolken, J. J. A molecular morphology of *Euglena gracilis* var. *bacillaris*. J. Protozool. 3:211-221, 1956.

164a. Wolken, J. J. Comparative study of photoreceptors. Trans. N. Y. Acad. Sci. 19:315-327, 1957.

165. Wolken, J. J. Photoreceptor structures. I. Pigment monolayers and molecular weight. J. Cellular Comp. Physiol. 48:349-369, 1956.

165a. Wolken, J. J. *In* Allen, M. B., ed. Comparative biochemistry of photoreactive systems. Academic Press, New York, 1960, p. 145-167.

165b. Wolken, J. J. Studies of photoreceptor structure. Ann. N. Y. Acad. Sci. 74:164-181, 1958.

165c. Wolken, J. J. The photochemical apparatus: its structure and function. Brookhaven Symp. Biol. No. 11:87-100, 1959.

166. Wolken, J. J. The structure of the chloroplast. Ann. Rev. Plant Physiol. 10:71-86, 1959.

166a. Wolken, J. J. The chloroplast and photosynthesis—A structural basis for function. Am. Scientist 47:202-215, 1959.

167. Wolken, J. J. and Mellon, A. D. The relationship between chlorophyll and the carotenoids in the algal flagellate, Euglena. J. Gen. Physiol. 39:675-685, 1956.

168. Wolken, J. J., Mellon, A. D., and Greenblatt, C. L. Environmental factors affecting growth and chlorophyll synthesis in *Euglena*. I. Physical and chemical. II. The effectiveness of the spectrum for chlorophyll synthesis. J. Protozool. 2:89-96, 1955.

169. Wolken, J. J. and Palade, G. E. An electron microscope study of two flagellates. Chloroplast structure and variation. Ann. N. Y. Acad. Sci. 56:873-889, 1953.

170. Wolken, J. J. and Schwertz, F. A. Chlorophyll monolayers in chloroplasts. J. Gen. Physiol. 37:111-121, 1953.

171. Wolken, J. J. and Shin, E. Photomotion in *Euglena gracilis*. I. Photokinesis. II. Phototaxis. J. Protozool. 5:39-46, 1958.

INDEX